Health Expenditure, Income and Health Status Among Indigenous and Other Australians

M.C. Gray, B.H. Hunter and J. Taylor

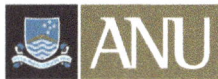

ANU
THE AUSTRALIAN NATIONAL UNIVERSITY

E PRESS

Centre for Aboriginal Economic Policy Research
The Australian National University, Canberra

Research Monograph No. 21
2002

ANU
E PRESS

Published by ANU E Press
The Australian National University
Canberra ACT 0200, Australia
Email: anuepress@anu.edu.au
Web: http://epress.anu.edu.au

Previously published by the
Centre for Aboriginal Economic Policy Research,
The Australian National University

National Library of Australia
Cataloguing-in-publication entry.

Health Expenditure, Income and Health Status Among Indigenous and Other
Australians

Includes index

ISBN 1 920942 15 7
ISBN 1 920942 14 9 (Online document)

1. Aboriginal Australians - Health and hygiene. 2. Torres Strait Islanders - Health and
hygiene. 3. Aboriginal Australians - Medical care. 4. Torres Strait Islanders - Medical
care. 5. Medical care, Cost of - Australia. I. Taylor, John, 1953- . II. Hunter, Boyd.
III. Title.

362.1089915

Designed by Green Words & Images (GWi)
Cover design by Brendon McKinley

Foreword

This monograph has its genesis in an approach made to the Centre for Aboriginal Economic Policy Research (CAEPR) by the Australian Institute of Health and Welfare (AIHW). CAEPR was asked to undertake an analysis of 1995 National Health Survey data as input to the AIHW's second report on expenditures on health services for Aboriginal and Torres Strait Islander people. This approach was made late in 1999, and agreement to undertake the work was completed early in 2000. The AIHW's report *Expenditures on Health Services for Aboriginal and Torres Strait Islander People, 1998–99* (AIHW cat. no. IHW 7) was published in 2001, but it did not include the CAEPR analysis. This delay was outside CAEPR's control and resulted from a series of unexpected delays in data acquisition and processing. This meant that CAEPR's analysis was only completed late in 2001; it was agreed by AIHW and the Office of Aboriginal and Torres Strait Islander Health in the Commonwealth Department of Health and Ageing that the CAEPR analysis should be published and widely disseminated as a late companion to the AIHW publication. The support of the Office of Aboriginal and Torres Strait Islander Health in facilitating this publication is gratefully acknowledged.

CAEPR's specific task was to analyse and report on health expenditures on Aboriginal and Torres Strait Islander people in comparison with expenditures on other Australians of similar socio-economic status. Two key relationships are explored—between expenditures and the distribution of equivalent family income, and between expenditures and health status. At one level, the findings extend the analysis in the report *Expenditures on Health Services for Aboriginal and Torres Strait Islander People* by J. Deeble, C. Mathers, L. Smith, J. Goss, R. Webb and V. Smith, published in 1998. In particular, access to 1995 National Health Survey (NHS) data provided an opportunity for more meaningful analysis of income relativities, with an added link to health status, because of the inclusion in the 1995 NHS of an Indigenous identifier for the first time.

This monograph is published in the CAEPR Research Monograph Series in part because it appears later than the second AIHW report, and in part because it utilises an established channel of publication which targets Indigenous interest groups, as well as the academic community and policy makers. Though written as a stand-alone document, its value is enhanced if read as a companion to the second AIHW report. As such, it reflects a positive outcome of collaboration between CAEPR and two government agencies (AIHW and the Office of Aboriginal and Torres Strait Islander Health in the Department of Health and Ageing), with important consultancy assistance also from the ABS.

I commend the monograph's authors, Matthew Gray, Boyd Hunter and John Taylor, for their perseverance and research commitment when faced by unanticipated hurdles, and believe this research outcome, while a little late, will be of great value in the general area of Indigenous health policy and research.

Professor Jon Altman
Director, CAEPR
August 2002

Acknowledgments

Preparation of this report was commissioned by the Australian Institute of Health and Welfare (AIHW) and conducted under its guidance, as well as that of the 2nd Expenditure Report Steering Committee convened by the Office of Aboriginal and Torres Strait Islander Health (OATSIH) in the Department of Health and Ageing. Accordingly, considerable institutional input and assistance require acknowledgment. First of all, we are indebted to John Goss and Justine Boland of the AIHW for their interest and assistance in pursuing this analysis, and for perceptive comments on various drafts. Second, thanks are due to Helen Evans and Alison Killen of OATSIH for their sustained interest and for facilitating publication. Valuable comments on drafts from steering committee members were provided by the National Aboriginal Community Controlled Health Organisation, AIHW, and OATSIH. Others who provided helpful comment on the report included Beverly Sibthorpe and John Deeble from the National Centre for Epidemiology and Population Health, Steven Kennedy of the Australian Bureau of Statistics (ABS) and Roger Jones of the Centre for Aboriginal Economic Policy Research (CAEPR). Particular mention should also be made of the technical assistance provided by Stephen Carlton, Tenniel Guiver, Tony Lloyd, and Daniel Smith of the ABS in accessing unit record data from the 1995 National Health Survey. A draft of this paper was presented in the CAEPR seminar series, and again to the Economics and Indigenous Australian Health Workshop held at the University of Melbourne between 29 and 30 November 2001. Our sincere thanks to all the participants of those two forums. Any errors in the paper are the sole responsibility of the authors. Editorial assistance was kindly provided by Hilary Bek and Frances Morphy.

Contents

7. Conclusion

37

Appendices

List of figures and tables

Figures

Tables

Abbreviations and acronyms

ABS	Australian Bureau of Statistics
AIFS	Australian Institute of Family Studies
AIHW	Australian Institute of Health and Welfare
AR–DRG	Australian Refined – diagnosis related group
ATSIC	Aboriginal and Torres Strait Islander Commission
BEACH	Bettering the Evaluation and Care of Health
CAEPR	Centre for Aboriginal Economic Policy Research
CHINS	Community Housing and Infrastructure Needs Survey
CHIP	Community Housing and Infrastructure Program
DRG	diagnosis related group
GP	general practitioner
HREOC	Human Rights and Equal Opportunity Commission
HIPP	Health Infrastructure Priority Project
ICD	International Classification of Diseases
NAHS	National Aboriginal Health Strategy
NATSIS	National Aboriginal and Torres Strait Islander Survey
NCEPH	National Centre for Epidemiology and Population Health
NHS	National Health Survey
OATSIH	Office of Aboriginal and Torres Strait Islander Health
OECD	Organisation for Economic Cooperation and Development
PBS	Pharmaceutical Benefit Scheme
SLA	statistical local area
SRS	simple random sampling
SMR	standardised morbidity ratio

Executive summary

Using data from the 1995 NHS this report asks the question—what is the relationship between income, health expenditure and health status for the Indigenous and non-Indigenous populations? The analysis seeks to measure differences in health expenditure and reported health status between the Indigenous and non-Indigenous populations holding income level constant. This is important to the extent that income is seen as an indicator of ability to address the need for health expenditure, and as a factor in influencing health status. A previous study of the relationship between income and expenditure on health found that Indigenous people were in receipt of expenditure equivalent to others in a similar economic position. As for the relationship between income and Indigenous health status, no previous analysis has ever been undertaken. The expectation, though, from the international literature is that income and health status are positively related.

The key findings from this study were as follows:

- The data refer to Indigenous and non-Indigenous populations in non-sparsely settled areas only. As such, they do not claim to be representative of the situation Australia-wide, especially in regard to the Indigenous population. They reflect the circumstances of the 82 per cent of the Indigenous population located in non-sparsely settled areas.

- Notwithstanding the above, use of 1995 NHS data enables direct comparison between Indigenous and non-Indigenous Australians with respect to the links between income status, health expenditure and health status for the first time.

- Previous studies have only managed to estimate the relationship between income status and expenditure. For this the Henderson measure of equivalent income was employed.

- The present study indicates the importance of developing a range of measures of equivalent income, as substantial differences in relative income distribution are evident depending on the measure used. In order to simplify the analysis, people are ranked by income and classified into quintiles (i.e. an income group with 20 per cent of the population).

- Per capita health expenditure on Indigenous people living in non-sparsely settled areas is estimated to be $2734 in 1995 (i.e. only for the comparable areas of health expenditure examined). This is some $500 higher than the estimate of $2277 for non-Indigenous people.

- This expenditure gap between Indigenous and non-Indigenous people is not statistically significant. However, if spending on hospitals is excluded (due to unreliability), then Indigenous per capita expenditure is significantly lower ($930 compared with $1351).

- As found in other Western countries, non-Indigenous health expenditure is significantly higher for low-income or poorer families. In contrast, no significant relationship between income and per capita health expenditure was found for Indigenous people.

- According to the NHS measure of health service utilisation (whether used a health service in the previous two weeks), Indigenous people were found to use health services much less than other Australians despite experiencing higher rates of morbidity and mortality.

- In line with expectation, the NHS data reveal a significantly positive relationship between non-Indigenous income and reported health status.

- While Indigenous people were more likely to report being in poor or fair health than other Australians for each income group, more striking was the lack of significant difference in self-reported health status between low and high-income Indigenous families.

- This lack of relationship remained even after adjusting for age difference between the low and high-income Indigenous families.

Equity issues: comparing like with like

A good deal of attention is devoted in this report to establishing appropriate measures of income for the purpose of comparing Indigenous and non-Indigenous outcomes. Because the family circumstances of Indigenous Australians are so different from that of other Australians, simply comparing families with similar income is misleading. For example, if spending (either in health or other expenditure) enhances the well-being of all family members, then expenditure can be said to provide 'public goods' within the family. Alternatively, expenditure may provide purely private benefits for a particular family member, depending on whom (or even on what) the money was spent. The approach adopted is to use several measures of equivalent income which cover the range of possible assumptions about family circumstances from all expenditure being on public goods (raw income) to the other extreme where all expenditure is on private goods (per capita income). As with previous analysis of Indigenous health expenditure, the Henderson measure of equivalent income is also used.

Examination of the overall distribution of Indigenous income illustrates why it is important to consider alternative definitions of income. While Indigenous people are over-represented in the 20 per cent of Australian families with the lowest income (the bottom quintile), there are large differences between the alternative measures of income. For example, over one-half of Indigenous families are in the bottom quintile of per capita income compared with less than 30 per cent in the bottom quintile of raw family income. Furthermore a detailed analysis of Indigenous income indicates that there is substantial re-ranking within income quintiles, with as many as one-third of families changing income group when different income measures are used.

Estimating per capita health expenditure by income—method and data issues

In principle, the best way to obtain estimates of per capita health expenditure by income is to collect individual-level information on the usage and associated costs of health services, income, Indigenous origin, age and gender. Unfortunately no such Australian data exist, and we are therefore forced to combine estimates of utilisation rates of health services (for each income and demographic group) from the 1995 NHS with the average costs of medical services estimated from a variety of administrative and survey data sources. The following health services are included in the estimates of per capita health expenditure by equivalent income:

- out-of-hospital visits to general practitioners or medical specialists;

- other health professional services;

- admitted hospital patient services;

- non-admitted hospital patient services;

- prescription medications; and

- over-the-counter medications.

The 1995 NHS contains information on 53 751 Australians of all ages and is representative of those living in all areas. It is important to note, however, that due to concerns about the quality of some of the responses from Indigenous participants who do not speak English at home, the estimates in this report exclude Indigenous and non-Indigenous people living in sparsely settled areas. In total, 539 records from survey participants in such areas were excluded, of which 461 were Indigenous. Thus, the final Indigenous sample upon which all NHS data contained in this report are based amounted to the 1753 respondents in non-sparsely settled areas. The estimates show that the Indigenous sample was representative of 82 per cent of the Australia-wide Indigenous population.

One drawback of the 1995 NHS is its inability to separate health expenditure into private and public components. Unlike the 1989 NHS which asked about hospital utilisation in the previous twelve months, the 1995 NHS asked about hospital utilisation in the previous two weeks. As a consequence, there were insufficient reported visits to hospitals to provide for the estimation of private and public hospital utilisation rates by equivalent income. Furthermore the 1995 hospital data were found to be unreliable, being based on a handful of respondents, especially for the high-income Indigenous population.

Another important caveat is that, by estimating health expenditure via the utilisation of health services recorded in the NHS, an important element of public health expenditure is excluded from the analysis—spending on the provision of environmental health infrastructure.

Per capita health expenditure by income and Indigenous origin

Our estimate of per capita health expenditure for Indigenous people living in non-sparsely settled areas is $2734, which is around $500 higher than the estimate of $2277 for non-Indigenous people. However, the estimates of per capita health expenditure are quite variable, and this difference between Indigenous and other Australians is not significant. When the unreliable hospital data are excluded, per capita health expenditure on Indigenous people is estimated to be significantly lower than the non-Indigenous average ($930 and $1351 respectively).

The expenditure for each income group reveals a similar pattern, with Indigenous expenditure being higher, albeit insignificantly higher, before hospital data are excluded. This pattern is reversed when the focus is on non-hospital related expenses, with Indigenous expenditure being significantly lower irrespective of family income.

Consistent with the international literature, non-Indigenous health expenditure is, on the whole, significantly higher for low-income or poorer families. In contrast, there is no significant relationship between income and per capita health expenditure for Indigenous people.

In order to test whether this apparent anomaly is due to the reliability of aggregate estimates of per capita expenditure, the utilisation of health services is estimated for each income group. The same story is replicated with no significant relationship between income and utilisation for the Indigenous population, except perhaps when the per capita income measure is used. For the non-Indigenous population, there is a significant relationship for most measures of income (except the Henderson measure) with lower-income families being slightly more likely to have used a health service in the previous two weeks. On average, the levels of utilisation reveal that, whatever the family income, Indigenous people use health services much less than other Australians, despite experiencing higher mortality and morbidity.

Health status by equivalent income

In line with expectations, the NHS data reveal a significantly positive relationship between non-Indigenous income and reported health status. While Indigenous people were more likely to report being in poor or fair health than other Australians for each income group, the more interesting finding was the lack of significant difference in self-reported health status between low and high-income Indigenous families. Why should there be a different relationship between the Indigenous and non-Indigenous populations? One possibility is that there is a difference in the patterns of self-assessed health status between Indigenous and non-Indigenous Australians, although this runs counter to research findings to date for populations in non-remote areas. Another possibility is that differences in self-reported health status may be partly explained by difference in age structure between the two populations, given that health status generally declines for older people. To test for this, the data are age-standardised. This involves adjusting the Indigenous statistics using the age distribution of the non-Indigenous population as weights. When this is done, there is still no relationship evident between income and health status for the Indigenous population, except when the measure of raw income is used.

Discussion

Difference in the relationship between health expenditure and income for Indigenous and other Australians is at least partially attributable to the more uniform poor health status of the former across income groups. While the lack of any association between income and Indigenous health status may simply reflect poor data quality, both in terms of income and self-assessed health status, there are two other possible explanations for the results: the Barker and social exclusion hypotheses.

The Barker hypothesis refers to the idea that adult mortality and morbidity may be related to foetal and infant life. In particular, it is proposed that diseases such as coronary heart, type 2 diabetes, central obesity and hypertension (all highly prevalent among Indigenous adults) originate through adaptations that the foetus makes to under-nutrition. Given the trajectory of Indigenous economic development since the 1960s, it is arguable that the present generation of Indigenous people in the upper income quintiles are far more likely than their non-Indigenous counterparts to have been exposed to the trifecta of low birthweight, poor nutrition and childhood disease that can reap such havoc in later life.

An alternative explanation to the Barker hypothesis is that current income is probably a poor proxy for socio-economic status among Indigenous people because they have been, and continue to be, socially excluded from mainstream society, irrespective of income. The main implication of both the Barker and social exclusion hypotheses (albeit for different reasons) is that it will take a long time to address the health deficits among Indigenous Australians. While the Barker hypothesis implies that there is a need to concentrate health expenditure on mothers and babies, the social exclusion hypothesis emphasises the need for ongoing support from both the community and governments across the entire lifecycle.

1. Background issues

While the broad profile of ill health and excess mortality among Indigenous Australians is well documented, research on determinants remains relatively undeveloped. Nonetheless, sufficient insight exists to place an emphasis in explanation on the compound effects of overall low socio-economic status, including low income. This is in line with theoretical trends generally in social epidemiology in which biological pathways between psychosocial stress and ill health are seen as explanatory (Berkman & Kawachi 2000; Kawachi, Kennedy & Wilkinson 1999; Marmot & Wilkinson 1999). Within this paradigm, persistently low levels of life expectancy among Indigenous Australians would be viewed as a product of their entrenched position at the bottom of the socio-economic hierarchy.[1]

One aspect of this focus in recent years has been to explore the linkages between Indigenous health and institutional arrangements for health care delivery and expenditure. Thus, in considering Indigenous health development, issues to do with interactions between minority Indigenous and majority non-Indigenous institutions are increasingly to the fore. Conceptually, these fall within a framework of what has been described as the 'new public health', which stresses the contribution of social justice, social action, power and access to resources as key components of Indigenous health outcomes.

To date, this redirection has generated insights at three levels. The first is at the scale of discrete communities where the focus has been on measuring the effects of improved environmental health infrastructure and identifying institutional impediments to achieving this (Torzillo & Kerr 1991). At a more macro-level, the consequences of control over health policy and its delivery have been explored in the context of Australian federalism, and at a comparative international scale (Bartlett & Legge 1994; Hogg 1992; Kunitz 1990). Finally, the consequences of low socio-economic status for health status are increasingly being examined at both the individual and group levels (Deeble et al. 1998; Gray & Broughton 2001; Hogg 1990; Hunter 1999, 2000a, 2001). The present analysis falls firmly within the last category, although some overlap with the first is also achieved through examination of the relationship between income and health expenditure using micro-level data.

Healthy expenditure?

Previous analysis of the amounts spent on health services for and by Aboriginal and Torres Strait Islander people found that the per capita level was about eight per cent higher than that spent for and by other Australians. Government health expenditure on Aboriginal and Torres Strait Islander people was found to be 47 per cent higher than on other Australians (Deeble et al. 1998). To assess whether this represented an equitable allocation, it was noted that relative expenditure fell well short of implied levels of Indigenous need, given that death rates for the Indigenous population were around three times the national average. By comparing government expenditure on Indigenous and other Australians in the lowest income group, the conclusion was drawn that Indigenous people were in receipt of expenditure equivalent to others in a similar economic position, but their worse health status was not adequately reflected. In further pursuit of a 'needs-based' formula for resource allocation, comparative crude death rates have been applied as a proxy for morbidity to argue for an additional 27 per cent increase in total expenditures on Indigenous health (NCEPH 2000).

While excess mortality provides a rough indication of need, it offers no guidance as to the cost-effectiveness of resource allocation for treating differentially prevalent morbidity. Such an approach would focus on 'capacity to benefit' and, ideally, a formulation would be based on equal expenditures for the same medical conditions. However, as Deeble et al. (1998: 52) point out, while such a calculation should be possible, it would not be the only criterion for allocating government expenditures since equality by medical need would be sufficient only if all services were publicly provided to all people without charge. This is not the case.

The amount of money spent on the health of each individual is comprised of expenditure by government (public health expenditure) and private health expenditure. It is an observed fact that the balance of these expenditures on individuals varies such that a positive correlation exists between income levels and the proportion of the population with private health insurance (Deeble et al. 1998: 57). Furthermore, people with higher income tend to have more out-of-pocket payments through schemes like the Pharmaceutical Benefit Scheme (PBS). The significance of this observation is seen in the quite different income distributions of the Indigenous and non-Indigenous populations. In 1996, Indigenous family incomes were on average 32 per cent lower than non-Indigenous family incomes. *Ipso facto*, dependence on public expenditure for access to health services is greater among Indigenous people.

This report asks the question—what is the relationship between income, health expenditure and health status for the Indigenous and non-Indigenous populations? The analysis draws out differences in expenditure between the Indigenous and non-Indigenous population holding income level constant. This is important to the extent that income is seen as an indicator of ability to address the need for health expenditure.

Unlike the analysis for the Australian population as a whole presented in Deeble et al. (1998), changes in the questions on the 1995 NHS mean that it is not possible to separate expenditure into private and public components, and therefore the analysis in this report deals only with total health expenditure. In spite of this limitation, the analysis remains of policy value since there is no existing analysis of health expenditure by income for the Indigenous population.

Data sources

This report presents an analysis of per-capita health expenditure by income for Indigenous and non-Indigenous Australians based on the utilisation of a range of health services as set out by questions asked in the 1995 NHS. This survey was conducted on a multi-stage area sample of private dwellings and a list sample of non-private dwellings (hotels, motels etc.). Hospitals, nursing homes and convalescent homes were excluded from the survey, as were prisons, reformatories and single quarters of military establishments. A base sample size approximating one-third of one per cent of the population was initially chosen. Inclusion of the Indigenous status question on the survey form yielded a total of 1100 Indigenous persons. To enhance the reliability of data for the Indigenous population an additional 1100 Indigenous respondents were sought. In doing this, the ABS used a sampling methodology which ensured that Indigenous respondents were representative of the population from which they were drawn. Thus, the total NHS sample included 2168 people who identified as being of Aboriginal or Torres Strait Islander origin.

It is important to note that, due to concerns about the quality of some of the responses from Indigenous participants who do not speak English at home, NHS estimates exclude Indigenous and non-Indigenous people living in those areas identified by the ABS as being sparsely settled, as in these areas non-English speakers predominate.[2] In total, 539 records from survey participants in such areas were excluded, of which 461 were Indigenous. The final Indigenous sample for this report is based on 1536 Indigenous respondents in non-sparsely settled areas for whom there were valid data on household income. The weighted estimates for 1995 show that this Indigenous sample was representative of 82 per cent of the Australia-wide Indigenous population (ABS 2000c: 34).

The utilisation data from the NHS include 'out-of-hospital visits to general practitioners or medical specialists', 'other health professionals', 'admitted hospital patients', 'non-admitted hospital patients', 'prescription medications', and 'over-the-counter medications'. In establishing expenditures based on these data, consideration was given to the age and sex patterns of utilisation which were found to vary significantly. It should be noted that changes to NHS questions on the utilisation of health services mean that the estimates of hospital utilisation are very unreliable for the Indigenous population. In the 1990 NHS, hospital utilisation was measured over the 12 months prior to the survey, whereas in the 1995 NHS the reference period was only the prior two weeks. Given the small size of the Indigenous sample and the low frequency of hospital visits, there are insufficient cases to ensure statistical reliability. Note that when converting these utilisation data to estimates of national expenditure, the amounts spent on each health service reported in the NHS were obtained from AIHW using a composite of administrative and supplementary survey data aggregated across different sources for varying geographic levels.

A caveat

By estimating health expenditure via the utilisation of health services as reported in the NHS, an important, and often overlooked, element of public health expenditure is excluded from the analysis—spending on the provision of environmental health infrastructure. Despite a well-established link in the international public health literature between living conditions and population health, few Australian studies have detailed the relationship between specific environmental problems and particular illnesses among Indigenous Australians. One pioneering study in this field is based on identifying nine healthy living practices for one community in the Anangu Pitjantjatjara lands (Pholeros et al. 1993). While this research indicated that improvements in environmental infrastructure can lead to specific improvements in health status, the key finding showed that this depends on ensuring that appropriate institutional arrangements are in place.

In particular, it is essential that budgets make adequate provision for planning, design, supervision and maintenance of infrastructure, and that these actually occur. Among the reasons for a lack of such arrangements in the past, confusion over myriad responsibilities for service delivery and marginalisation of environmental health issues in the policy system has been highlighted.

The major government response to such inadequacies developed out of the National Aboriginal Health Strategy (NAHS) in 1990, which recognised an essential linkage between improved health outcomes and the provision of housing and infrastructure to acceptable minimum standards. Accordingly, funding allocations in the initial years of the NAHS primary health and environmental health programs included amounts directed at housing and infrastructure services within Aboriginal and Torres Strait Islander Commission's (ATSIC) Community Housing and Infrastructure Program (CHIP). However, a review of CHIP in 1994 identified a range of problems including a failure to address housing and infrastructure needs in a holistic way. Allied to this was the short-term nature of the program-based approach to funding, which required communities to structure housing needs to the CHIP program rather than the other way around.

Such criticism led to the establishment, in the same year, of the Health Infrastructure Priority Projects (HIPP) program to pilot new program delivery arrangements for the construction of Indigenous community housing and infrastructure in 58 sites. This has subsequently expanded, and in 1998–99 a total of $103 million was allocated via NAHS/ HIPP initiatives. Notwithstanding this environmental health expenditure, the 1999 Community Housing and Infrastructure Needs Survey (CHINS) found that fully one-third of the housing stock administered by Indigenous housing organisations in discrete communities remained in need of major repair or replacement (ABS 2000b:3). While part of the difficulty here is catch-up—given the legacy of previous neglect—the question of equity in regard to the adequacy of this public expenditure remains open.

Equity issues: comparing like with like

The ability of income to translate into better health depends, among other things, on the extent to which spending affects various family members and the amount of resources left over after various expenditures. For example, if spending (either in health or other expenditure) enhances the well-being of all family members, then expenditure can be said to provide 'public goods' within the family. Alternatively, expenditure may provide purely private benefits for a particular family member. Obviously, the relationship between income and expenditure depends crucially upon the proportion of public goods in household spending. Equivalent income measures control for the extent of consumption of public goods, which may vary with family size and composition. This was a feature of the previous analysis of Indigenous health expenditure which applied the Henderson measure of equivalent income to account for such issues (Deeble et al. 1998).

In testing for equity in health expenditure, it is necessary to compare observed health expenditures for Indigenous people with outlays on health for other Australians in the same income group. One constraint on establishing a precise comparison in the Deeble et al. (1998) analysis was the lack of data consistency. The problem was that information on Indigenous incomes was drawn from the 1994 National Aboriginal and Torres Strait Islander Survey (NATSIS), while data on non-Indigenous incomes were derived from the 1990 NHS.

In the present study, estimates of both Indigenous and non-Indigenous income and health service utilisation are derived using data from the same source. This is possible for the first time because the 1995 NHS included a question on Indigenous status. The availability of a common source of data ensures that the following analysis has a higher level of methodological consistency than was previously possible. Perhaps, most importantly, the availability of Indigenous utilisation data from the 1995 NHS provides for the calculation of standard errors on the estimates, thereby enabling the significance of differences in expenditure by income to be tested. Once again, this represents an advance on previous analysis of expenditure by income.

The 1995 NHS data also provide income data adjusted using the ABS's version of the simplified Henderson equivalence scales. Since any one of a number of equally plausible equivalence scales may be chosen, it is necessary to consider whether our results are affected by using alternative scales. The equivalence scales used in this report therefore cover the full range of possibilities from all expenditure being on public goods (raw income) to the other extreme where all expenditure is on private goods (per capita income).

Expenditure, income and health status

A further advantage of the 1995 NHS data is the capacity they provide to extend the analysis of the relationship between income status and expenditure, and to explore the links between these factors and health status for both the Indigenous and non-Indigenous populations. While such analysis is desirable, legitimate concerns surround the extent to which a suitable measure of health status is available from the NHS to enable meaningful comparison between Indigenous and non-Indigenous populations. In effect, the exclusion of sparsely settled areas from the NHS sample partly resolves this issue, as argued below.

This same dilemma regarding the potential usefulness of self-assessed health status was raised and extensively investigated subsequent to the release of results from the 1994 NATSIS (Cunningham, Sibthorpe & Anderson 1997). This survey (as well as the 1995 NHS) asked a global question on self-assessed health status as follows:

> In general, would you say that your health is excellent, very good, good, fair or poor?

Given objective evidence of higher Indigenous morbidity and mortality, an apparent similarity in self-reported rates of poor to fair health among the Indigenous and non-Indigenous respondents in the NATSIS (around 17 per cent each) suggests that differential thresholds for reporting poor or fair health were being applied. If this were so, it would potentially undermine the utility of data on self-assessed health status as a proxy for comparison of health needs between groups. However, as Cunningham, Sibthorpe & Anderson (1997: 26) have pointed out, expected differences in self-assessed health status were evident between the two populations after accounting for age structure. This variation was sufficient to suggest that the limitations of the data did not override their utility for comparative purposes. Further evidence from the NATSIS also supports the utility of responses to the global question on self-assessed health status. This is drawn from the fact that individuals who reported that they had a long-term health condition were significantly more likely to report poor or fair health than those who indicated that they had no long-term condition (Cunningham, Sibthorpe & Anderson 1997: 18).

While, in principle, the utility of the global question may be accepted, one concern remains to be overcome. This is based on the observations that the level of reported poor or fair health in the NATSIS was markedly lower for people who indicated that they did not speak English as their main language, and that other estimates for this group also displayed a large degree of response error (Cunningham, Sibthorpe & Anderson 1997: 19–21). Similar error among Indigenous respondents whose main language was not English was found in the ABS evaluation of Indigenous data quality issues in the 1995 NHS (Gray 1997). Indeed, it was concern over data quality for this group that led to their exclusion from the calculation of final published estimates. Thus, by focusing the sample on respondents from non-sparsely settled areas, residual doubt about the utility of the global question on self-assessed health status is largely overcome.

2. Indigenous health status in perspective

Infant mortality

The infant mortality rate is used internationally as one of the key indicators of community health. It is defined as the number of infant deaths (deaths of children less than one year of age) for every 1000 live births. Among Indigenous Australians there was an exceedingly high rate of infant mortality of around 100 infant deaths per 1000 live births—recorded as recently as the mid-1960s. In subsequent years, there was a steady and precipitous decline to around 26 per 1000 by 1981, with much of this due to improvements in post-neonatal mortality. While further improvement in infant survival also occurred during the 1980s and 1990s, this has been less impressive, with Indigenous infant mortality rates remaining consistently around two and a half times the Australian average. Consequently, about seven per cent of Indigenous male deaths and eight per cent of Indigenous female deaths occur to people less than one year-old. This compares with only one per cent of all deaths among all other infants (Cunningham & Paradies 2000). The latest available data from the ABS indicate an infant mortality rate among Indigenous infants of 14.1 per 1000 live births compared with 5.7 per 1000 live births among all infants (ABS 2000a: 75).

For Indigenous Australians, the initial drop in infant death rates coincided with improvements in community infrastructure and the development, in the 1970s, of intensive Indigenous health programs and services. However, this medical intervention is not the only factor leading to declines in infant mortality. While access and equity issues remain important in terms of the delivery of health care services to Indigenous Australians, further significant improvements in infant survival are also reliant on a decrease in the proportion of low birthweights which, in turn, is heavily correlated with nutritional issues, smoking rates, and the socio-economic status of mothers. In 1995–96, the proportion of low birthweight babies (less than 2500 grams) born to Indigenous mothers was almost twice that of babies born to non-Indigenous mothers (12.4 per cent compared with 6.2 per cent). Such low birthweight babies are less likely to survive, and those who do survive are more likely to have worse health early in life, and perhaps even in adulthood.

Life expectancy

In 1973, the Australian government gave itself 10 years to raise the standard of health of Indigenous people to the level of that of the rest of the population. Almost 30 years later, Indigenous life expectancies remain stuck at around 20 years lower than the rest of the Australian population. The first reasonable national estimates of Indigenous mortality were obtained from 1981 and 1986 Census data and revealed life expectancies to be around 56 years for males and 64 years for females. Also apparent was a relative lack of mortality variation between the states and territories, although life expectancies were lowest in regions with the most remote and rural communities, a situation that has persisted. However, a pattern of relatively high death rates at all ages, but especially in middle adulthood between 30 and 50 years, was found to be universal. Once again, this feature has shown little sign of subsequent abatement. While analysis of 1991 Census and mortality data indicated a slight improvement in overall survival prospects, data from the 1996 Census point to a slight worsening of overall mortality, with no change in male life expectancy but with female life expectancy falling below 64 years. One consequence partly associated with this differential mortality is that the Indigenous population has a much younger age profile with a median age in 1996 of 20 years compared with 34 years for the non-Indigenous population.

Leaving aside problems of identification of Indigenous people in official records, there is sufficient evidence to suggest that underlying age-specific death rates vary among Indigenous populations living in different parts of the country. The lowest life expectancies (53.7 years for males and 58.9 years for females) are found in the western half of the continent in Western Australia, South Australia and the Northern Territory. In the eastern half, life expectancies are somewhat higher (59.2 years for males and 63.6 years for females). Not surprisingly, the western jurisdictions closely match the distribution of regions which have persistently displayed the greatest socio-economic disadvantage against indices incorporating measures of housing adequacy, educational attainment, employment status and income status.

The most striking feature is the overall lack of progress in raising Indigenous life expectancies, given that survival chances for the total Australian population have undergone marked improvement over the period for which reliable Indigenous estimates have been available. More poignant is the fact that the level of mortality observed for Indigenous males at the end of the twentieth century is equivalent to that recorded for all Australian males at the beginning of the century. Among females, the comparison is similarly discouraging, with life expectancy for Indigenous females currently hovering around a level last recorded for females generally in 1920. This lack of steady improvement in life expectancy, despite declines in infant mortality, is a different demographic phenomenon compared with that of Indigenous peoples in New Zealand and North America, and it persists because of much higher rates of Indigenous Australian adult mortality.

Mortality—rates and causes

Estimation of the true national level of Indigenous mortality remains constrained by incomplete vital registration. While the ABS now publishes reported Indigenous death statistics for all states and territories, most detailed tabulations, and certainly those used for trend analysis, are based on information from the Northern Territory, Western Australia and South Australia only. This is based on an assessment of the completeness of recording from a comparison of registered deaths in each state and territory against an estimate of expected deaths. Overall, in 1999, a total of 1980 Indigenous deaths were registered. This was more than twice the number that would have been expected if the age-specific death rates of the total Australian population were experienced throughout the Indigenous population.

Using data for the Northern Territory, Western Australia and South Australia, age-specific death rates were higher than for other Australians at all ages, but especially among those aged between 25 and 64 years (Cunningham & Paradies 2000: 30). For example, between the ages of 35 and 44 years, the ratio of Indigenous to non-Indigenous mortality rates is 6.9 for males and 7.8 for females (ABS and AIHW 1999: 132). While it is difficult to establish detailed trends in Indigenous mortality, owing to changes over time in the coverage of Indigenous deaths in vital statistics, there appears to have been a decline in age-specific death rates since 1994 in all age groups except for 15–24 and 45–54 years (ABS 2000a: 75). Overall, it remains the case that a high proportion of registered Indigenous deaths occur among young people. In 1999, the national median age at death for Indigenous people was 53 years, some 25 years less than the median age at death of all Australians (ABS 2000a: 74).

A good deal is now known about the immediate causes of ill-health and mortality among Indigenous Australians. Across all primary categories of the International Classification of Diseases (ICD9), relative risk for both Indigenous males and females remains notably higher than for other Australians. Most disparities, however, are concentrated around diseases of the circulatory system, external causes, and malignant neoplasms, while a relatively high incidence of respiratory diseases, endocrine diseases and diseases of the digestive system is also present. Together, these causes account for more than two-thirds (69 per cent) of the excess deaths among Indigenous people.

According to the most recently available data from deaths registration, diseases of the circulatory system are the leading cause of death among the Indigenous population, accounting for 31 per cent of all cases in 1999. Primary among these is ischaemic heart disease, responsible for 56 per cent of all recorded deaths in this category, followed by cerebrovascular disease (stroke) accounting for 19 per cent of deaths.

The second leading cause of death (16% of all Indigenous deaths) is external causes (including accidents, assault and intentional self-harm). By contrast, external causes are responsible for only seven per cent of deaths among the total population. Significantly, the median age at death for external causes is much lower among Indigenous people (28 years)—more than 10 years less than among the rest of the population.

Malignant neoplasms (cancers) account for about one-seventh of Indigenous deaths (14%). The most common of these (responsible for around 50 per cent of cases) are malignant neoplasms of the trachea, bronchus and lung. Diseases of the respiratory system and endocrine, nutritional and metabolic diseases are the next main causes of death (8% and 7% respectively). Among the latter, diabetes is responsible for as much as 87 per cent of all cases. Consequently, excess mortality due to diabetes is more than eight times the expected level if age-specific rates of the total population are applied. Diseases of the digestive system represent the final leading cause of death category among Indigenous people, accounting for five per cent of all deaths. This prevalence is four times that observed among the total population. The major contributor to Indigenous mortality within this category is liver disease.

Morbidity

Data on hospital separations are often used as indicators of morbidity. However, as Deeble et al. (1998: 46) point out, these are imperfect measures as high rates may reflect not only serious morbidity but inadequate primary care or specialist services (especially in areas where Indigenous people are the predominant population). Low rates, on the other hand, may simply be the result of difficulties of access. In either event, the decision to hospitalise is often subjective and based on different perceptions of the need for hospital care on the part of doctors and health workers.

Cunningham and Beneforti (2000) have produced a major study of Indigenous and non-Indigenous hospital statistics that has greatly assisted in the analysis of morbidity. Despite implementation of the National Aboriginal and Torres Strait Islander Health Information Plan, as well as a series of framework agreements involving the federal, state and territory governments, inadequate identification of the Indigenous population within hospital records remains a major constraint for analysis. As a consequence, comparisons of the Indigenous population with other Australians using hospital statistics will underestimate the true differences between the two populations.

Notwithstanding under-reporting, and after adjusting for age differences, almost twice as many hospital separations were reported in 1997–98 for those identifying as Indigenous than would have been expected if they had experienced the same rates as the total population. Higher rates of Indigenous hospitalisation were also reported in the Northern Territory, Western Australia and South Australia, although the extent to which this reflects jurisdictional differences in the completeness of Indigenous identification in hospital records is unknown. At the same time, hospitalisation rates also appear to be highest in remote areas (more than twice the non-Indigenous rate), while rates for Indigenous people in rural and metropolitan centres were still between 1.5 and 1.7 times higher than for the rest of the population.

One striking observation in the Cunningham and Beneforti analysis, which is of direct relevance for the present study, is that fully 98 per cent of separations identified as Indigenous in 1997–98 occurred in public hospitals, compared with only 68 per cent of non-Indigenous separations. This partly reflects the under-identification of Indigenous patients in private hospitals, although it is consistent with the pattern of highest public health spending among the lowest income groups.

By far the largest reason for hospitalisation among those identified as Indigenous in 1997–98 was regular and repeat visits for dialysis. A sense of the much greater burden of hospital care due to dialysis for Indigenous people compared with the rest of the population is provided by the standardised morbidity ratio (SMR) for this cause of 6.7 for males and 11.2 for females.[3] Use of SMRs as a guide to other major causes of Indigenous hospitalisation reveals relatively high ratios (>2.0) for endocrine/nutritional and metabolic disorders, infectious diseases, respiratory diseases, and diseases of the skin and subcutaneous tissue. However, as a proportion of all Indigenous separations, complications of pregnancy and childbirth, respiratory diseases and injury dominated for women, while the most common causes for men were respiratory diseases and injury.

Reported illness and health status

The 1994 NATSIS yielded information on self-reported recent illness and long-term health conditions. This has been summarised by the ABS (1996) and provided the basis for establishing a morbidity profile in Deeble et al. (1998). While the distinction between recent and long-term conditions was also sought in the 1995 NHS, it is considered that a combination of these conditions provides the most useful information from the NHS, given the somewhat artificial distinction between them, certainly in the minds of many respondents (ABS 1999: 5).

The majority of Indigenous and non-Indigenous males and females in every age group reported at least one recent or long-term condition in the 1995 NHS. Overall, more than three-quarters of Indigenous people (76%) reported a recent or long-term condition, although this was lower than the proportion of non-Indigenous people (86%). However, since the proportion of people reporting such conditions increases with age, true comparison requires age adjustment. This reveals that the reported levels of illness were equivalent among Indigenous and non-Indigenous respondents, although cross-cultural comparison of self-reported conditions is problematic.

As in the NATSIS, diseases of the respiratory system were the most commonly reported types of condition by Indigenous people (37% of reported cases) but, unlike in the NATSIS, a much greater incidence of diseases of the nervous system was reported (34 per cent of cases). These were also the two most commonly reported disease categories for the rest of the population. Typical respiratory conditions included asthma, sinusitis, bronchitis, emphysema and influenza, with little variation in prevalence observed across age groups. As for diseases of the nervous system, these referred mostly to eye and hearing problems, which both increased markedly with age.

Among specific conditions, asthma was more commonly reported for Indigenous people than for non-Indigenous people in every age group, and was particularly prevalent among children and youth below the age of 25 years. More striking was that the reporting of diabetes was seven to eight times higher for Indigenous people between the ages of 25 and 55 years. Overall, diseases of the circulatory system were reported by 15 per cent of Indigenous people. While this was less than for the non-Indigenous population (21%), hypertension was notably higher among Indigenous people, especially in young adult to middle age groups (25–55 years) where reported levels were three times higher than for the rest of the population.

Contrary to what might be expected from morbidity statistics and continuing high levels of mortality, almost three-quarters (73%) of NHS Indigenous respondents reported their health status as 'good', 'very good' or 'excellent'. However, this was notably lower than the proportion of non-Indigenous respondents (83%). It is also the case that Indigenous males and females were far more likely than their non-Indigenous counterparts to report their health as 'poor' or 'fair' at all age groups, especially over the age of 25 years. Even though objective statistics might suggest greater difference between Indigenous and non-Indigenous self-assessed health status, the fact that some difference is evident is in itself significant, given that self-assessments may be affected by individual awareness and expectations about health, and factors such as differential access to health care and health information.

Health risk factors

It has long been recognised that Indigenous people experience relatively high exposure to risk factors that are strongly associated with a variety of chronic, preventable and non-communicable diseases. While sometimes reported as 'lifestyle' factors, as in the case of smoking or alcohol consumption, not all health risks stem from behavioural decision making. Also important are more structural influences, such as living conditions and the means to improve nutrition.

The idea that Indigenous community housing should be designed, constructed and maintained to support healthy living practices is now firmly embedded in government policy. The National Indigenous Housing Guide includes a range of design and functionality guidelines aimed at ensuring access to adequate functional housing, clean water, and safe disposal of refuse and waste as a means of disease prevention (Commonwealth of Australia 1999). In the meantime, the reality of many Indigenous communities around the country remains a substantial backlog of need in the provision of healthy housing and infrastructure. Difficulty in overcoming this need is compounded by populations that are not only growing rapidly in size, but are also increasingly dispersed in distribution.

Using census-derived normative measures of overcrowding, it has been calculated that 14 865 Indigenous households in non-improvised dwellings (16% of the total) were overcrowded in 1996 (Jones 1999). In addition, 1883 Indigenous families and 1310 individual Indigenous adults were recorded in improvised dwellings. Overall, this translates into almost 35 000 additional bedrooms required to eliminate overcrowding. At the same time, the 1999 CHINS revealed that 30 per cent of the 20 400 dwellings included in the survey required major repairs or replacement, thereby highlighting the persistent problem of depreciating stock and need for asset management. In addition, only 14 per cent of the 1291 communities in the survey were connected to town water supplies, with most dependent on bore water or alternative sources, especially the smaller communities of less than 50 persons. Even among the larger communities of more than 50 persons, almost half (44%) of those not connected to town supplies had no water treatment facility. This pattern of infrastructure provision is mirrored in sewerage systems, with only seven per cent of communities using a town system and the majority reliant on septic or other systems. A total of 69 small communities had no sewerage system.

It has long been recognised that poor diet and nutritional status are strongly associated with cardiovascular disease and diabetes, but malnutrition also forms part of the general complex of reduced resistance to infectious and other disease, and may engender its own morbidity profile, as in the form of osteoporosis, dental caries, gall bladder disease, nutritional anaemias, digestive tract disorders and diet-related cancers. It is also the case that nutritional disorders are relatively high among Indigenous populations. One recent study, for example, estimates that as much as 20 per cent of Aboriginal children in the Top End of the Northern Territory are malnourished (Ruben & Walker 1995).

Anthropometric measures, such as weight adjusted for height and age, can provide useful indicators of nutritional status and associated risk of long-term ill health. For example, underweight pregnant mothers often give birth to underweight babies, while being underweight in childhood (wasting) can lead to slower physical growth and failure to thrive. On the other hand, being overweight is a risk factor for a number of health conditions in adult life, such as diabetes and heart disease. The 1995 NHS provides information on self-reported height and weight for adults aged 18 years and over. This suggests that Indigenous adults were more likely than other adults to be obese (16% compared with 11%) and less likely to be of acceptable weight (29% compared with 42%). This observation is deliberately cautious because of the high non-response of Indigenous respondents to NHS questions on weight and height (22% compared with 9%). As for nutritional indicators for children, these are available for those aged between seven and 15 years from the NATSIS and have been analysed by Cunningham and Mackerras (1998). Compared with Australian standards, Indigenous children are more likely to be underweight or obese and less likely to be of acceptable weight. This is true of both sexes, although the discrepancies are greatest in rural areas and least in capital cities, especially in regard to wasting.

Tobacco smoking is a well-known risk factor for a number of major causes of mortality including heart disease, lung disease and cancers of various types. It has also been linked to low birthweight. According to the 1995 NHS, 51 per cent of Indigenous adults aged 18 years and over living in non-remote areas indicated that they currently smoked, compared with only 23 per cent of non-Indigenous adults. The size of this gap was similar for both males and females, although male smoking levels were generally higher. Excess alcohol consumption is also a major health risk factor and, although Indigenous adults are less likely than other adults to drink alcohol, they are more likely to do so at hazardous levels. Thus, the 1995 NHS reports that 51 per cent of Indigenous adults did not consume alcohol, compared with 44 per cent of all other adults. However, of those who consumed alcohol, 23 per cent of Indigenous people did so at medium to high levels of risk, compared with only 10 per cent of other adults.

Information is available via the 1999 CHINS on aspects of physical access to health services. This survey covered all discrete Indigenous communities (1291) across Australia embracing a population of 109 000, which approximated 27 per cent of the total estimated Indigenous population in 1999. While the majority of such communities are located in sparsely settled areas and are excluded from the NHS sample, the CHINS data do refer to a wider area than this, and therefore have some relevance to the interpretation of NHS results.

Many communities (69%) were located more than 100 kilometres from the nearest hospital, with smaller communities more likely than larger ones to be distant from hospitals. On a reported population basis, this comprised 54 per cent of the population in discrete communities—a total of 58 860 persons. While only 53 per cent of communities remote from hospitals had access to emergency air medical services, these tended to be the larger communities, and so 86 per cent of the population in such communities had access to emergency air medical services. Again, on a population basis, 90 per cent of the population in discrete communities were located within 25 kilometres of a first-aid clinic. However, lack of transport can impede service usage, and so the CHINS also measured the frequency with which health workers visited communities that were more than 10 kilometres from a hospital. This revealed that only nine per cent of such communities had daily access to a doctor, 54 per cent had weekly or fortnightly access, 22 per cent had access monthly or less frequently, and 15 per cent had no access. These data support the findings from case studies that indicate that a lack of physical access to health services remains a constraint on improved health outcomes (McDermott, Plant & Mooney 1996).

3. Comparing like with like: analysis by income

An essential step in comparing like with like is to adjust family income for family size and composition in order to take into account differences in the costs of living. This is particularly important when comparing the per capita health expenditure of Indigenous and non-Indigenous Australians by income level due to substantial differences in the size and structure of households between the Indigenous and non-Indigenous populations.

There is an ongoing and unresolved debate regarding appropriate equivalence scales for use in Australia (Saunders 1994). In the present analysis, the major challenge is to ensure that the distinctive circumstances of Indigenous people are taken into account in any reform of widely used equivalence scales (Altman & Hunter 1998).

Use of the 1995 NHS as a common data source for income equivalence and estimates of expenditure enables the calculation of all-important standard errors on the estimates of health expenditure by income. However, this introduces certain constraints on the analysis, and a discussion of these is provided.

Estimating access to resources using equivalent income

One important dimension of the capacity of Indigenous people and families to pay for health expenditure is family or household income. In order to calculate the resources available for improving health, one must appreciate the overall demands on resources within a family or household. There is no consensus on how this should be done, and several standard techniques exist to adjust family income to allow for the different number and characteristics of family members—that is, to apply an equivalence scale.[4] Note that while equivalence scales are standard tools in poverty analysis, they will be used in this report to provide an indication of the overall access to resources within families, some of which could potentially be spent on health services.

As indicated above, the NHS provides income data adjusted using the ABS's version of the simplified Henderson equivalence scales. However, this is only one of several scales available and, as noted, there is an ongoing controversy about the precise specification of equivalence scales. This revolves around the nature and extent of economies of scale in families or households—the smaller the proportion of expenditure on items which display economies of scale, the more justifiable it is simply to divide family or household income by the number of people it supports (Guobao, Richardson & Travers 1996). When income levels are very low, a high proportion of expenditure is on food, basic clothing, cooking fuel and certain health expenditures. Given that each of these varies directly, and quite closely, with the number of people in the family, it may make it appropriate to give each person a similar weight by focusing on per capita income. In contrast, where so-called 'public goods' (i.e. where a certain expenditure improves the well-being of all residents and not only the person consuming the resources) are important, such as in various categories of health expenditure, more account needs to be taken of potential economies of scale implicit in the equivalence scales. At the extreme, raw income measures implicitly assume that extra family members cost no more to maintain than the first person. While this assumption is obviously untenable, it provides a useful bound on possible assumptions about economies of scale.

The point to note from this sensitivity analysis is that the relationship between health expenditure and income is likely to be distorted through measures of income which do not adjust for the number and age of people living off that income.[5] The per capita equivalence scales overestimate the needs of larger families in comparison with smaller families (De Vos & Zaidi 1997). In contrast, the use of raw income underestimates the needs of such families. The equivalence scales used in this paper cover the majority of possible assumptions about household costs, ranging from there being no extra cost to additional persons living in the family to there being no economies of scale in people living together. Given the preponderance of larger families in the Indigenous population the analysis of Indigenous health expenditure may be particularly sensitive to the type of income measure used.

Another tension implicit in choosing the appropriate equivalence scale for Indigenous income units is that the definition of the appropriate unit of analysis is not obvious in the Indigenous context (Altman & Hunter 1998). The widely used Henderson equivalence scales may be appropriate for a nuclear family, but it is more difficult to rationalise their use when Indigenous households can be characterised as having: compositional complexity; porous social boundaries and large size; extended families resident in one or more dwellings; households being subject to considerable fluctuation; and small, multi-generational core(s), dissolving and reforming in developmental cycles (Altman et al. 1997). Hunter and Smith (2000) have argued that focusing on households, rather than families, makes comparisons between Indigenous and non-Indigenous populations particularly problematic, especially when using the standard ABS definitions. Because of the conceptual difficulties in measuring income in a cross-cultural context, this paper uses a variety of equivalence scales on family income to capture the likely sensitivity of results to the underlying assumptions about economies of scale and access to resources.[6]

The income measures are calculated for income units (i.e. families) using four equivalence scales: raw income, the Henderson scale, the new OECD scale and per capita income.[7] Raw income is simply the sum of income of family members. The other income measures adjust for the size and composition of families by dividing this raw income by their respective equivalence scale.

While Henderson's scale has been the standard measure for equivalent income in Australia since the mid-1970s, there is increasing criticism of the robustness of the resulting estimates (Henderson 1975; Saunders 1994; Travers & Richardson 1993). Accordingly, two extra measures of equivalent income are included to explore the feasible range of access to resources. However, Henderson's scale does have the advantage that it is the only scale to attempt to control for extra costs incurred by working or looking for a job. This adjustment is likely to be particularly important when comparing estimates of Indigenous and other Australians, given the enormous disparity in employment rates between these groups (Taylor & Hunter 1998).

Another equivalence scale widely used in international studies of poverty is the OECD scale. This paper uses the new or modified OECD scale, which gives a weight of one to the first adult, 0.5 to the second and subsequent adults, and 0.3 to all dependants (see De Vos & Zaidi 1997 for further details of the history of the OECD equivalence scales).

The last income measure used is per capita family income. This is calculated by dividing the raw income by the number of people in a family. The advantage of using these four income measures is that they cover the range of possibilities of economies of scale and access to resources. As discussed above, raw income and per capita income provide the extreme bounds of possible assumptions, with the Henderson and new OECD measures falling somewhere within these bounds. While the Henderson and new OECD scales probably provide more feasible estimates of access to resources, the sensitivity analysis needs to test whether our results are robust to all possible measures. Note that Fig. 3.1, and all subsequent analysis, reports the equivalent income measures in descending order of implicit economies of scale: raw income, the new OECD scale, the Henderson scales and per capita income.[8]

Income quintiles for these four different measures of income were estimated from the 1995 NHS separately for the Indigenous and non-Indigenous components of the population (Fig. 3.1). Each estimate is ranked according to its place in the overall distribution of the respective measures of equivalent income in the 1995 NHS. That is, the income quintiles used in this paper are measured for the Australian population using NHS 1995 data. Accordingly, the non-Indigenous distribution, which dominates the overall income distribution, is even, with 20 per cent being in each quintile.

Fig. 3.1   Distribution of equivalent income, Indigenous families

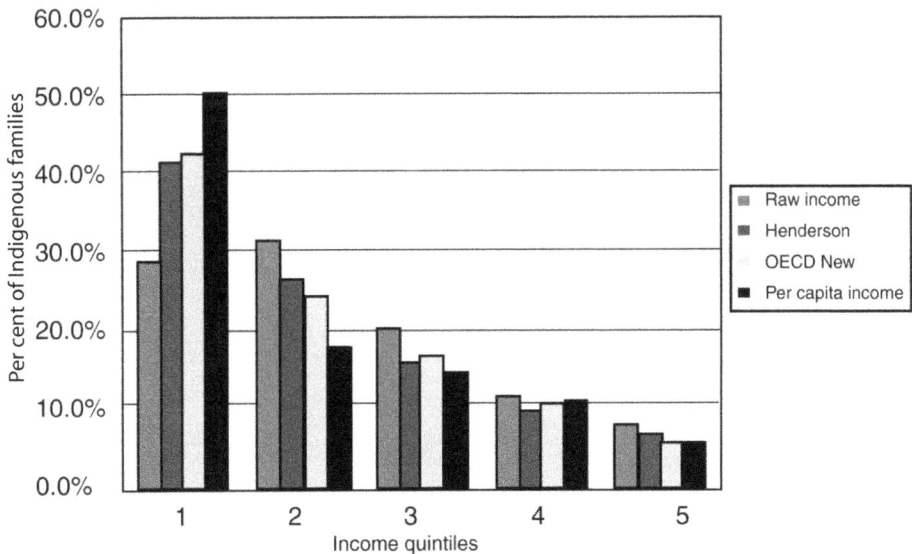

Source: NHS 1995, Appendix tables B1, B3, B5, and B7.

In line with Deeble et al. (1998), Fig. 3.1 illustrates that Indigenous people are disproportionately concentrated in the low income groups. As this earlier study only reported the distribution of equivalent income using a simplified Henderson scale, it is useful to compare this with other income distributions. One obvious point to make is that the per capita measure of equivalent income is even more concentrated in the low income group (at least, the bottom quintile). For example, per capita income is about 10 percentage points more likely to classify Indigenous families in the lowest quintile than the Henderson measure. On the other side, Henderson classifies over 10 per cent more of the Indigenous population in the bottom quintile than does raw income. Notwithstanding this, the overall shape of the distribution is similar, with most of the differences occurring in the first and second quintiles. The top two quintiles have very similar numbers of Indigenous families in all four income distributions.

Even though some of the overall income distributions in Fig. 3.1 do not differ much for the various measures of equivalent income, there are substantial reclassifications of families between the respective scales. Large families are more likely to be in the high quintiles of raw income, irrespective of living circumstances. While such families will tend to be reclassified in the lower income groups with the other equivalence scales (especially the per capita measures), other family types will be reclassified into higher income groups. The fact that Indigenous families are almost twice as likely to have a sole parent than other families with children complicates the comparisons between Indigenous and other Australian families (Daly & Smith 1998a; Daly & Smith 1998b). The extent of reclassification of family income depends crucially upon the number of children in the family and the assumption made about the relative costs of children and adults for the respective equivalence scales (Hunter, Kennedy & Smith 2001).

The age profiles of the various income groups can affect the interpretation of an income-based analysis.[9] For example, if low income groups include disproportionate numbers of older people, who would be more likely to be sick irrespective of their income status, then improvements in health as one moves up the income distribution may be driven as much by demographic factors as by differential access to resources or information. A brief perusal of age profiles by income reveals that this is the case for almost all measures of equivalent income used in this report, especially for the non-Indigenous population. The exception is per capita income, where the bottom quintile group has relatively few people aged 55 years or more (four times fewer than in the second quintile). The likely reason for this is that per capita income tends to re-rank small families at the end of the lifecycle (i.e. where the children have left home) into high-income quintiles compared with large families with many dependants. Whatever the reason, the fact that the age profile differs across income measures means that if the following analysis points to consistent differentials, irrespective of the equivalence scale, then it is possible to rule out that the analysis is driven by demographic factors.

Detailed analysis of the NHS income data indicates that there is substantial re-ranking of families or income units across income quintiles, with as many as one-third of families changing income group when different equivalence scales are used (Hunter, Kennedy & Smith 2001). Given the substantial reclassification of income groups for both Indigenous and non-Indigenous populations, it would be surprising if the analysis of health expenditure was not sensitive to the choice of equivalence scales. Exploration of these effects provides for a more sophisticated treatment of income than was possible in Deeble et al. (1998) and yields greater insight into the relationship between income, health status and expenditure.

Estimating per capita health expenditure by income—method and data issues

Method

In principle the best way to obtain estimates of per capita health expenditure by income is to collect individual-level information on the usage and associated costs of medical services, income, Indigenous origin, age and gender. Unfortunately no such Australian data exist, and we are therefore forced to combine estimates of utilisation rates of health services from the 1995 NHS with the average costs of medical services estimated from a variety of administrative and survey data sources.

The method used involves merging onto the 1995 NHS, at the level of each individual record, estimates of the average cost of medical services. This produces, for the individuals in the NHS survey, estimates of the expenditure associated with the medical services they used in the two weeks prior to the survey. Using the estimated expenditure and information on each respondent's equivalent income, it is straightforward to estimate average per capita health expenditure for Indigenous and non-Indigenous Australians.

There are two sources of sampling errors associated with the estimates of per capita health expenditure. First, there is sampling error associated with the estimates of utilisation rates of health services from the 1995 NHS. Second, there are errors in the estimates of the average cost per medical service. The standard errors of the estimates of the utilisation rates are calculated using the 'jackknife' method.[10] Unfortunately, no information is available on the standard errors of the estimates of the average cost per medical service. Given that such costs are estimated from data which relate to a substantial proportion of the total population, it is reasonable to assume that the sampling variability from this source is extremely small. Notwithstanding, the standard errors of the estimates of per capita health expenditure presented in this paper provide a lower bound estimate.

The method of estimation of per capita health expenditure by income differs in a number of respects from that used in a previous analysis of this relationship. Deeble et al. (1998) estimated total and government health expenditure by age and gender, and then allocated this expenditure across equivalent income quintiles using differences in average rates of utilisation of health services for income groups.[11] The analysis by income group was only done for the total Australian population. Overall Indigenous public health expenditure was then compared with the estimates for the total Australian population for the respective income groups. The argument was made that Indigenous people are predominantly in the lowest income group and that per capita health expenditure should be compared with government health expenditure on the lowest income group for the total Australian population.

As outlined above, the estimates presented in this report are constructed by combining estimates of the average costs per medical service (estimated primarily from administrative data sources) and utilisation rates estimated from the 1995 NHS. The analysis is conducted at the level of the individual, and so no allocation of total health expenditure across income groups is required. The main advantage of the approach used in this report is that it allows standard errors on the estimates of health expenditure by income. As will become apparent when the results are presented, the standard errors are very high, and conclusions drawn about differences in health expenditure which ignore the standard errors may be grossly misleading.

Data

The 1995 NHS contains information on 53 751 Australians of all ages and is representative of those living in all areas. There is information on the rates of utilisation of a variety of health services but no information on the costs of these services. The NHS also contains information on income and a range of demographic variables. The following health services are included in the estimates of per capita health expenditure by equivalent income:

- out-of-hospital visits to general practitioners or medical specialists;

- other health professionals;

- admitted hospital patient;

- non-admitted hospital patient;

- prescription medications; and

- over-the-counter medications.

The range of medical services included in the estimates of expenditure is determined by the questions asked in the 1995 NHS. More information on the definition of each medical service is presented in Appendix A.

As indicated above, the analysis of health expenditure by income uses four equivalence scales to derive separate measures of equivalent income:

- raw family income;

- Henderson;

- OECD (new); and

- per capita income.

Income quintiles for these four different measures of income were estimated from the 1995 NHS separately for the Indigenous and non-Indigenous components of the population. Each family's income is ranked using the overall distribution of equivalent income in the 1995 NHS. Given that the number of Indigenous families in some of the higher quintiles is quite small, it is necessary to aggregate the top four quintiles to enhance the reliability of the estimates.[12] The numbers of people in the respective quintiles are provided for each measure of equivalent income in Appendix B.

In the interests of transparency (i.e. to ensure that the results are replicable), Appendix C provides detailed breakdowns of all the costs per service for medical services used in this report. As discussed, these estimates were provided to CAEPR by AIHW and are derived from a variety of administrative data sources. Where possible, the estimates of cost per medical service are estimated according to Indigenous origin, gender and age group. The level of disaggregation in the estimates of cost per service varied according to what is feasible, given the administrative data available (see Table 3.1 for details of the level of disaggregation for each category of medical service). Where no disaggregation is possible, it is necessary to assume that the cost per service is identical across age groups, gender and Indigenous origin. The medical services for which disaggregated cost data are available are admitted patients, visits to general practitioners and specialists, and prescription medications.

It is important to estimate cost per medical service by as detailed a gender, age and Indigenous origin breakdown as possible due to differences in the average cost per service by demographic characteristics. The importance of this is illustrated by the differences in the estimated costs per service for admitted patients; these vary from $478 per day in hospital for Indigenous males aged 75 plus years to $900 per day in hospital for non-Indigenous females.

Table 3.1   Level of disaggregation of costs per medical service for each type of medical service

Medical service	Level of disaggregation of estimates of cost per service
Admitted patients	By Indigenous origin, gender and 10-year age groups
Non-admitted patients	Single estimate for population as a whole
Prescription medications	By Indigenous origin, gender and 10-year age groups
Over-the-counter medications	Single estimate for population as a whole
Other health professionals	Single estimate for population as a whole
General practitioners and medical specialists – out of hospital	By Indigenous origin and gender. For age groups 0–44 and 45+ for the Indigenous population and 10-year age groups for the non-Indigenous population.

Note: Unfortunately, it was not possible to further disaggregate the out-of-hospital estimates for the Indigenous population because it is based on a relatively small sample size (see endnote 13).

The medical services for which disaggregated cost data are available cover 78.7 per cent of all health expenditures included in this analysis. The inaccuracies introduced by the aggregated nature of the estimates of over-the-counter medications, non-admitted patients and other health professionals will be relatively minor. It is worth stressing that no information was provided on the standard errors associated with the estimates of cost per medical service. The standard errors, for at least some of the service types, are likely to be quite large. For example, the cost per visit to a GP for the Indigenous population is based upon information from 2000 Indigenous patient encounters. This means that the number of patient encounters in each of the gender and age groups is small for the Indigenous population.[13]

As already noted, unlike the analysis for the Australian population as a whole presented in Deeble et al. (1998), it is not possible to separate expenditure into the private and public components. There are several reasons for this, all associated with the quality of information available from the 1995 NHS. First, due to changes in the questions about rates of medical service utilisation between the 1989 and 1995 NHS, it is not possible to estimate government health expenditure by equivalent income quintile. The main change is that the 1989 NHS asked about hospital utilisation in the previous twelve months, whereas in 1995 the NHS asked about hospital utilisation in the previous two weeks. This means that there are not enough reported visits to private hospitals to allow utilisation rates of private and public hospitals by equivalent income to be estimated.

Second, the proportion of expenditure on prescription medications that is privately funded versus the proportion publicly funded is determined by several factors. Prescription medications listed on the PBS receive a government subsidy.[14] Prescription medications which are not listed on the schedule of PBS-approved drugs receive no subsidy, and therefore all costs are borne privately. Clearly, in order to estimate public versus private funding on prescription medications, it is crucial to separate medications according to those listed on the PBS schedule and those not listed on the PBS schedule. This is not possible using the 1995 NHS because it classifies medications according to their Anatomical Therapeutical Category, and this cannot be mapped onto PBS and non-PBS categorisation.

There are major advantages to the method used in this report to estimate per capita health expenditure by income. First, it allows standard errors to be calculated for the estimates. This is absolutely critical when interpreting the estimates of health expenditure per capita for the Indigenous population for whom the sample sizes are small. Second, it gives an accurate reflection of per capita expenditure for the sample used rather than applying the rates to aggregate data. This of course means that the estimated per capita expenditure will differ from the estimates of aggregate expenditure.

4. Per capita health expenditure by income and Indigenous origin

Our estimate of per capita health expenditure for Indigenous people living in non-sparsely settled areas is $2734, which is around $500 higher than the estimate of $2277 for non-Indigenous people. However, the estimates of per capita health expenditure are quite variable, particularly for the Indigenous population, for whom the standard error on the estimate of per capita expenditure is $334. While the estimates for the non-Indigenous population are also variable, the standard errors are smaller ($50). This means that the estimate of per capita health expenditure on Indigenous people is not statistically different from the estimate for the non-Indigenous population (at the 95 per cent confidence level).

The high standard errors, particularly for the Indigenous population, result primarily from the unreliability of hospital data in the 1995 NHS. The relative rarity of hospital visits means that very few Indigenous respondents reported using a hospital in the two weeks before the survey. Consequently, standard errors on the hospital expenditure are very high, and estimates of health expenditure including hospital expenditure are unreliable.

When hospital usage is excluded, per capita health expenditure on Indigenous people is estimated to be much lower than the non-Indigenous average ($930 and $1351 respectively). The standard errors are much smaller—$64 and $11 for the Indigenous and non-Indigenous populations respectively—and there is statistical evidence that Indigenous health expenditure is significantly lower than that for other Australians, at least for some categories of expenditure.

High variability in hospital utilisation rates, combined with the fact that hospital visits are, on average, much more expensive than other medical services, means that this category of expenditure makes up a high proportion of total health expenditure. The high degree of variability in the hospital expenditure is a function of the fact that a very small proportion of the sample had visited a hospital for health-related reasons in the two weeks prior to interview. Some insight into this issue can be gained by looking at the numbers of the sample with health expenditure of more than $1000 in the two weeks prior to the survey. For the Indigenous population in the income quintiles two to five, there are 13 respondents who had health expenditure of more than $1000 in the two weeks prior to the survey, and a maximum health expenditure of $9147. There is a similar pattern for the non-Indigenous sample, although the larger sample size means that the problem is much less severe. Detailed information on the distribution of health expenditure by equivalent income is presented in Appendix B.

Table 4.1, which presents the estimates of per capita expenditure by equivalent income quintile for the non-Indigenous population, highlights a number of important issues.[15] First, there is a large amount of variation in estimated per capita health expenditure across the different measures of equivalent income. For example, the estimates of expenditure for the lowest quintile vary between $2735 using the raw family income, $2500 using the new OECD scale, $2316 using the Henderson equivalence scale, and $1892 using the per capita income scale. This dramatic variation in the estimates of expenditure by equivalent income for the different equivalence scales highlights the importance of the equivalence scale used and the need to conduct a sensitivity analysis for this type of analysis.

In general, the point estimates of per capita health expenditure show that expenditure has a negative relationship with equivalent income. For example, using the new OECD equivalence scale, for the lowest income quintile (quintile one) per capita expenditure is estimated to be $2500. It is $1982 for quintile two, $1678 for quintile three, $1511 for quintile four, and $1467 for quintile five. While expenditure is estimated to be larger for lower equivalent incomes for all of the equivalence scales, the standard errors are high, meaning that care needs to be exercised when interpreting these results.

Whether there are statistically significant differences in health expenditure between income groups can be formally tested using the following:

$$test\ statistic = \frac{E_1 - E_2}{\sqrt{SE(E_1)^2 + SE(E_2)^2}}$$

where E_1 and E_2 are the estimated expenditure of income groups one and two respectively and $SE(E_1)$ and $SE(E_2)$ are the standard errors of the estimates of E_1 and E_2. The denominator is simply the standard error of the difference between two random variables from simple random sample (see Appendix D). In conventional hypothesis tests, the 95 per cent confidence interval of an estimate is the point estimate plus or minus 1.96 times the standard error. Therefore, in order for there to be statistically significant differences in estimated per capita expenditure, the absolute value of the test statistic must be greater than 1.96.

For example, the new OECD scale expenditure estimates for income quintiles three and five respectively are $1678 and $1467, a difference of $211. The test statistic is 2.76, which is greater than the critical value of 1.96, and therefore we can conclude that there is a statistically significant difference at the 95 per cent confidence level. Similarly for the raw family income, the Henderson measure and per capita income, expenditure for income quintile three is significantly higher than for income quintile five with test statistics of 5.38, 1.97 and 8.08 respectively. Note that there are only three pair-wise comparisons in Table 4.1 for which income was not significantly negatively related to health expenditure: the differences between the fourth and fifth quintiles of Henderson and OECD income measures, and the difference between the first and second quintiles of the per capita income distribution.

Table 4.1   Per capita health expenditure ($ p.a.) by equivalent income, non-Indigenous population

	Raw family income		Henderson		New OECD		Per capita income	
Income quintile								
1	2735	(148)	2316	(133)	2500	(124)	1892	(96)
2	1930	(62)	1808	(69)	1982	(69)	2085	(57)
3	1627	(50)	1749	(64)	1678	(58)	1916	(50)
4	1552	(44)	1665	(41)	1511	(45)	1861	(49)
5	1261	(46)	1598	(42)	1467	(49)	1374	(45)

Note: The standard errors of the estimates of expenditure are presented in parentheses.

Given the relatively small numbers of Indigenous respondents in the top income quintiles, the estimates need to be further aggregated to allow comparisons between Indigenous and other Australians. Table 4.2 presents estimates of per capita health expenditure by equivalent income for the Indigenous and non-Indigenous populations for two income groups: the first income quintile, and income quintiles two to five combined. By grouping quintiles two to five together, the number of Indigenous respondents in the income groups was increased to an acceptable level.

Table 4.2   Per capita health expenditure (including hospital expenditure) by broad income group and Indigenous origin

	Raw family income		Henderson		New OECD		Per capita income	
Income quintile								
Indigenous expenditure ($ p.a.)								
1	3029	(786)	2404	(521)	2656	(627)	2114	(396)
2 to 5	2212	(406)	2434	(533)	2280	(443)	2689	(643)
Non-Indigenous expenditure ($ p.a.)								
1	2735	(148)	2316	(133)	2500	(124)	1892	(96)
2 to 5	1597	(51)	1704	(54)	1660	(56)	1808	(51)

Note: The standard errors of the estimates of expenditure are presented in parentheses. The per capita health expenditure is calculated across the same range of medical services as used in Table 4.1. The qualification that it includes hospital expenditure is made to distinguish it from the next table, which excludes such expenditure.

Unfortunately, the standard errors are still large for the Indigenous population, and it is not possible to draw any conclusions about the relationship between income and per capita expenditure. As with the overall estimates of Indigenous health expenditure, there is too much variability within income groups to identify whether genuine differences exist between the income groups.

The standard errors for the non-Indigenous estimates are also quite large. However, it is possible to conclude that for the raw family income, Henderson and new OECD equivalence scales, expenditure is higher for the lowest income quintile than for higher income groups (quintiles two to five). There is no statistically significant difference between income groups for the per capita equivalence scale. On the surface, this differs from the overall results for the more disaggregated income breakdown, which found that expenditure fell for all of the equivalence scales. This is an important point because it means that the aggregation of income groupings may hide underlying differences in expenditure by equivalent income.

In Table 4.3, further estimates of per capita health expenditure for low and high-income Indigenous and non-Indigenous Australians are shown, but this time excluding hospital expenditure.[16] The standard errors are now much lower. Health expenditure is substantially less for the Indigenous population than for the non-Indigenous population. The finding that non-Indigenous health expenditure (excluding hospital expenditure) is higher than for the Indigenous population is consistent with findings from another analysis of NHS data, which shows that Indigenous people are more likely to visit hospitals (outpatients and day clinics in particular) than to go to a GP or specialist (ABS/AIHW 1999: 74).

For the non-Indigenous population, expenditure is estimated to be significantly lower for the higher equivalent income groups when using the OECD, Henderson and raw family income equivalence scales. As in Table 4.2, there is no significant difference in expenditure across income groups for the per capita equivalence scale. This is probably driven by the fact that per capita scale changes the composition of families within the various quintiles. If large families have substantial economies of scale in health provision (i.e. they do not require as many services or as much health expenditure), then the fact that per capita scales tend to reclassify such families as low-income will depress the expenditure in the bottom quintile relative to the other income groups. This hypothesis is supported by the observation that expenditure on Indigenous people in the bottom quintile of per capita income is actually lower than for other Indigenous people, albeit not significantly lower.

In spite of the fact that estimates of health expenditure on Indigenous people are generally lower for high income groups, there is no statistically significant difference for any of the equivalence scales. However, the standard errors for the Indigenous estimates are still relatively large, and one should be careful that the results presented in Table 4.3 are not interpreted to mean that in reality there are no differences. Notwithstanding, if the focus is on the Henderson scale (as it was for Deeble et al. 1998), increasing the sample size is unlikely to render the difference significant, given that there is very little difference in expenditure between income groups. Also the fact that health expenditure is actually greatest in the high (Henderson) income group means that any significant statistic may not necessarily support Deeble et al.'s hypothesis of the relationship between Indigenous income and expenditure.

Table 4.3   Per capita health expenditure (excluding hospital expenditure) by broad income group and Indigenous origin

	Raw family income		Henderson		New OECD		Per capita income	
Income quintile								
			Indigenous expenditure ($ p.a.)					
1	1409	(185)	1175	(108)	1254	(147)	1021	(100)
2 to 5	1171	(112)	1197	(121)	1164	(106)	1249	(142)
			Non-Indigenous expenditure ($ p.a.)					
1	2527	(104)	2148	(92)	2283	(91)	1747	(72)
2 to 5	1494	(46)	1585	(49)	1526	(49)	1708	(48)

Note: The standard errors of the estimates of expenditure are presented in parentheses. The per capita health expenditure excludes hospital expenditure to distinguish it from the previous two tables, which include such expenditure.

A re-examination of Table 4.2 reveals there is no significant difference between Indigenous and non-Indigenous health expenditure in the respective income quintiles (e.g. comparing people in the bottom and higher quintiles separately). However, if poor quality hospital data are excluded in an attempt to reduce standard errors, then health expenditure on low-income Indigenous people is much lower than the expenditure on low-income non-Indigenous people, and these differences are statistically significant (Table 4.3). For example, using the Henderson scale the per capita expenditure on Indigenous people in the first quintile is estimated to be $1175 dollars, which is around $973 dollars less than the estimate of $2148 for non-Indigenous people in the same income group. The expenditure on higher-income Indigenous people is also uniformly lower than the expenditure on higher-income non-Indigenous people.

Therefore, by excluding hospital data from the calculation, we find that the difference in health expenditure between high and low income groups for Indigenous people is less substantial than the expenditure differential between Indigenous and other Australians. Income appears to add little to the analysis of health expenditure, either because income is poorly measured or because improvements in income are a relatively recent phenomenon among Indigenous people. In addition to the probable lags in improvements in health, and hence health expenditure, another aspect of the latter is that the experience of rapid upward social mobility may have greater pathological impact for Indigenous Australians (Sibthorpe 1988). Notwithstanding the limitations of income as an instrument to measure overall health expenditure, Deeble's (1998: ix) emphasis on analysing the relationship between public expenditure and income remains valid, given that many government payments are means tested.

On balance, it appears that there is little or no difference in Indigenous expenditure across income groups. This result is in stark contrast to the non-Indigenous results for whom high income groups tend to have lower health expenditure. One obvious explanation for this difference between Indigenous and non-Indigenous populations is that, while high-income Indigenous families appear to be as unhealthy as poorer Indigenous families

(Hunter 1999), there is a strong relationship between income and health outcomes amongst other Australian families (NHS 1992). The penultimate section of this paper returns to this theme by exploring the evidence in the 1995 NHS on the relationship between income and health for both Indigenous and non-Indigenous Australians.

5. Further information on the usage of health services by equivalent income

As discussed above, the estimates of per capita health expenditure by income group have a great deal of sampling variability and therefore high standard errors. We are therefore very constrained in our ability to determine whether there are genuine differences in health expenditure by income and whether there are differences between the Indigenous and non-Indigenous populations.

In an attempt to overcome this uncertainty, further analysis of usage of health services by equivalent income groups was conducted by focusing on those who reported no usage in the two weeks prior to interview. This is motivated in part by the fact that estimated proportions of people by Indigenous origin and income group will have less sampling error and therefore be more stable than the estimated total health expenditure by Indigenous origin and income group (Table 5.1). Another advantage of this shift in focus is that it provides a direct measure of Indigenous utilisation of health services, albeit one that does not capture the intensity of usage of respective services.

For the Indigenous population, there is no statistically significant relationship between the usage of health services and equivalent income, irrespective of the equivalence scale used.

A similar pattern is revealed for the non-Indigenous population. The only difference is that the proportion utilising health services in the lowest income group is significantly smaller than for the highest income group for the raw and per capita income measures. For example, using the raw family income groups, the proportion utilising health services rises from 51.5 per cent for the lowest income quintile to 54.3 per cent for the highest income quintile.

Table 5.1 Proportion who utilised health service in previous two weeks by broad income   group

	Raw family income		Henderson		New OECD		Per capita income	
Income quintile								
	Per cent of Indigenous expenditure ($ p.a.)							
1	44.2	(4.3)	39.0	(3.8)	38.3	(3.6)	35.0	(3.7)
2 to 5	40.1	(5.3)	39.5	(4.6)	45.1	(5.7)	49.5	(6.7)
	Per cent of non-Indigenous expenditure ($ p.a.)							
1	51.5	(0.7)	54.9	(0.8)	52.7	(0.7)	49.0	(1.0)
2 to 5	54.3	(0.8)	54.1	(0.8)	54.0	(0.8)	55.0	(0.7)

Note: The utilisation rates are based on the services described in Appendix A. The standard errors of the estimates of expenditure are presented in parentheses. See Appendix D for details of their calculations.

Note that there are substantial and significant differences between the Indigenous and non-Indigenous populations in the usage of health services. Low-income Indigenous people are much more likely than non-Indigenous people in the same income category to report not having used any health services (except for those classified using raw family income). The differential in usage of health services of Indigenous and other Australians is about 14 percentage points for the Henderson, new OECD and per capita scales, and is 7.3 percentage points for the raw family income scale. Given that less than 10 per cent of Indigenous people are aged 55 and over, compared with around 25 per cent of other Australians, demographic factors are likely to play a major role in explaining this differential. However, demographics cannot be the whole story because the proportion of older people (aged 55 years or more) in the bottom quintile of the per capita income measure is only marginally different between Indigenous and other Australians.

For the higher income groups, the estimated proportion of Indigenous people not using health services is also larger than for non-Indigenous people, but the differential is only statistically significant for the raw family income and Henderson scales. The relatively small difference between usage of health services between high-income Indigenous and other Australians (at least by this measure) is largely driven by the standard errors of the respective estimates, with non-Indigenous estimates being more reliable.

To summarise, in contrast to the earlier analysis, the level of Indigenous usage (or lack of usage) of health services across income groups appears to be similar to that of other Australians. Given the apparently weak relationship between income and the proportion without health expenditure, differences in the relationship between income and expenditure for Indigenous and non-Indigenous populations must be driven by the amount expended by those who spent some money on health.[17] In the next section we explore one possible explanation for this observation, in the context of establishing the relationship between self-assessed health status and equivalent income.

6. Health status by equivalent income

The analysis above suggests that for the non-Indigenous population a negative relationship exists between per capita health expenditure and equivalent income. In contrast, for the Indigenous population there is no evidence of a significant relationship between per capita health expenditure and equivalent income. Why should there be a difference in this relationship between the Indigenous and non-Indigenous populations? As far as per capita health expenditure is concerned, there are several factors that may be relevant. These can be separated into:

- differences in the met need for health and medical services (determined by both the number of medical conditions and the cost of treating those conditions);

- differences in access to medical services;

- differences in the costs of treating the same medical condition between Indigenous and non-Indigenous Australians; and

- differences in the knowledge and perception of need, which may be influenced by cultural and educational factors.

The differences in costs may be related to geographic location or differences in behaviour between the Indigenous and non-Indigenous populations.

An additional factor, which is considered here, is difference in self-assessed health status between Indigenous and non-Indigenous Australians. This is considered important since varying levels of self-assessed health status are assumed to reflect variation in the need for medical services. The analysis in this section uses information on self-assessed health status derived from the NHS global question: 'In general would you say that your health is: excellent; very good; good; fair or poor'.[18]

While this question enables only a crude measure of health status, research has found a high correlation between self-reported health status and standard measures of well-being, such as derived from the SF-36 survey instrument.[19] For the Indigenous population, Gray (1997) has also found a reasonable degree of correlation between responses to the global health question and the reporting of long-term health conditions, at least for those respondents in non-remote areas. Taken together, this research supports the use of the self-reported single global health status question as a valid indicator of real differences in health status.

Table 6.1 presents estimates of the proportion of the non-Indigenous population that reported having fair or poor health by equivalent income. As might be expected, given the findings from social epidemiological research (Kawachi, Kennedy & Wilkinson 1999), there is a marked decline in the proportion of those reporting fair or poor health as equivalent income increases. For example, for the new OECD equivalence scale, the proportion reporting fair or poor health falls from 25.3 per cent for the lowest income quintile to just 8.5 per cent for the highest income quintile. This is consistent with the differences in per capita health expenditure by equivalent income documented in Chapters 4 and 5. That is, at least some of the difference in health expenditure between high and low-income non-Indigenous Australians can be attributed to the better health status of the former.

Table 6.1   Per cent reporting fair or poor health by equivalent income, non-Indigenous population

	Raw family income		Henderson		New OECD		Per capita income	
Income quintile								
			Per cent reporting fair or poor health					
1	24.1	(0.6)	25.6	(0.7)	25.3	(0.6)	17.1	(0.7)
2	22.4	(0.6)	24.3	(0.7)	24.5	(0.7)	27.6	(0.7)
3	18.0	(0.7)	15.2	(0.5)	14.2	(0.6)	18.8	(0.5)
4	10.3	(0.4)	9.9	(0.5)	9.4	(0.5)	10.9	(0.4)
5	7.7	(0.4)	7.9	(0.4)	8.5	(0.5)	8.4	(0.4

Note: The standard errors are presented in parentheses.

Table 6.2 presents the analogous estimates of health status by broad grouping of equivalent income for the Indigenous and non-Indigenous populations. Given the relationship between age and health status, differences in self-reported health status may be partly explained by difference in age structure between the two populations, and so the data are age-standardised. This involves adjusting the Indigenous statistics using the age distribution of the non-Indigenous population as weights.

While age standardisation is a commonly used procedure, there are some doubts regarding the validity of its use in estimating Indigenous health status. There are two main concerns. First, selective mortality may introduce a systematic distortion into estimates of age-standardised health status. Second, the process of calculating equivalent income implicitly controls for the age structure of families by taking into account the number of dependants. However, the procedure for calculating equivalent income does not account for differences in the numbers of family members in old age groups who tend to have poorer health profiles. It is not possible to say conclusively whether or not age standardisation is a valid procedure in this case, and therefore both the age standardised and non-age standardised results are presented. This chapter concludes with a brief reflection on the value of age-standardising health status in the Indigenous context.

The results in Table 6.2 are consistent with those presented in Table 6.1. Thus, non-Indigenous people in high income groups tend to report significantly better health, although an exception to this generalisation arises in the per capita measure, with the high income group more likely to report poorer health. This result is largely driven by the aggregation involved in constructing Table 6.2. For example, non-Indigenous self-assessed health status in the fourth and fifth quintiles of per capita income is significantly better than in the first, second or third quintiles.

The non-age-standardised estimates for the Indigenous population reveal that there is little or no systematic relationship between income and health status. While low income groups are more likely to report poor or fair health (except for per capita income), the difference between income groups is not significant for any of the measures of equivalent income.

Consequently, the relationship between income and non-age-standardised health status can be characterised as weak, unsystematic and insignificant.

While this result is contrary to the general findings of research on the relationship between income and health status (Kawachi, Kennedy & Wilkinson 1999), it is supported by NATSIS data which revealed that Indigenous people in high income quintiles were just as likely to have a long-term health condition as other Indigenous people (Hunter 1999). Evidence of a low correlation between Indigenous health outcomes and labour force status is also available (Hunter 2000b).

The process of age standardising increases the percentage of the Indigenous population reporting poor health in the lowest income group. However, in general, the differences between income groups are still not statistically significant. Given the concerns expressed above about the extent of selective Indigenous adult mortality, this result should be viewed with suspicion. The only exception to this rule is for the raw family income scale.

Notwithstanding problems with the cross-cultural interpretation of health status, Table 6.2 also provides the opportunity to compare the health status of Indigenous and other Australians after controlling for income. The main effect of age standardising is to ensure that the reported health status of the non-Indigenous population is significantly better than that of the Indigenous population, irrespective of equivalence scale used, or income group. While there is less difference between the non-age-standardised health status of Indigenous and non-Indigenous people, there is a significant difference for most income groups at either the five or 10 per cent level. For example, in the bottom quintile of per capita income, Indigenous people are significantly more likely to report fair or poor health (24.7 per cent and 17.1 per cent respectively). Therefore, in spite of the difficulties with interpreting self-reported health status, there is evidence that Indigenous people are significantly less healthy than other Australians after the effect of income distribution is taken into account.

Table 6.2   Self-reported health status by broad income group and Indigenous origin

	Raw family income		Henderson		New OECD		Per capita income	
Income quintile								
Per cent of non-Indigenous population reporting fair or poor health								
1	24.1	(0.6)	25.6	(0.7)	25.3	(0.6)	17.1	(0.7)
2 to 5	17.5	(0.6)	17.6	(0.6)	17.2	(0.6)	19.1	(0.6)
Per cent of Indigenous populaiton reporting fair or poor health (not age-standardised)								
1	31.5	(4.0)	28.8	(3.5)	29.8	(3.4)	24.7	(3.4)
2 to 5	25.1	(4.7)	26.9	(4.2)	26.5	(5.1)	29.6	(6.1)
Per cent of Indigenous populaiton reporting fair or poor health (age-standardised)								
1	39.9	(4.2)	36.4	(4.7)	37.4	(4.1)	30.7	(3.9)
2 to 5	27.6	(3.2)	29.7	(4.0)	29.4	(4.4)	33.4	(5.6)

Note: The standard errors are presented in parentheses.

The potential biases introduced by age standardisation are investigated further by examining estimates of self-assessed health by five-year age group for the Indigenous and non-Indigenous populations (Table 6.3). Overall, Indigenous people are more likely to report their health status as being poor or fair than other Australians. Interestingly the difference is smallest for very young and very old people. It is probably not surprising that a similar percentage of Indigenous and non-Indigenous youth indicate that they consider their health to be poor or fair. This is suggested by the arguments reviewed in Chapter 2 that poor health is the cumulative consequence of prolonged exposure to risk factors, the consequences of which are not realised in self-reported health status for some years.

It is worth noting that the reported health status of the Indigenous population converges towards that of other Australians at the oldest ages. This convergence is a result of non-Indigenous people reporting poorer health in the older age groups, rather than a change in self-reported health status for Indigenous people. Indeed, it surprising that Indigenous people aged over 75 are about 10 percentage points less likely to report having poor or fair health status than are Indigenous Australians aged in their 50s and early 60s. It is difficult to explain why reported Indigenous health status appears to improve slightly after a person turns 50 years old.

Table 6.3 Per cent of age group whose self-assessed health status is poor or fair by age groups and Indigenous status

	Indigenous (1)	Non-Indigenous (2)	Difference (1)-(2)
Age group			
15–19	11.7	8.2	3.6
20–24	16.0	9.3	6.8
25–29	25.4	9.2	16.2
30–34	27.9	9.7	18.1
35–39	20.5	10.5	10.0
40–44	34.5	11.2	23.3
45–49	33.5	14.3	19.2
50–54	52.9	17.7	35.2
55–59	52.7	24.4	28.4
60–64	57.2	27.2	29.9
65–69	49.6	29.2	20.4
70–74	49.8	35.9	13.9
75 +	44.2	41.1	3.1

One reason might be found in the much higher adult mortality rates for Indigenous people, with those surviving to 'old age' tending to be genetically predisposed to better health. That is, the high rates of adult mortality among Indigenous people are selective and tend to make their health status look particularly good amongst older age groups. The process of age-standardising Indigenous statistics can distort comparisons between Indigenous and other Australians, as this process gives a higher weight to the responses of older Indigenous people on the grounds that they are under-represented relative to the rest of the population.

In summary, differences in the relationship between health expenditure and income for Indigenous and other Australians are at least partially attributable to the more uniform poor health status of the former across income groups. This may be one reason why those Indigenous Australians reporting higher incomes, with presumably more adequate access to (personal) resources, still require relatively substantial health expenditure.

7. Conclusion

As the information base for profiling Indigenous health outcomes and proximate causes is progressively expanded, the indications of high absolute and relative morbidity and mortality remain unchanged, as do reported levels of exposure to risk factors that are strongly associated with a variety of chronic, preventable and non-communicable diseases. From a policy perspective, one element of the health complex that lends itself most directly to intervention is the level of expenditure (both public and private) on health and medical services. Previous analysis of the distribution of such expenditure noted that total health spending per capita was higher for Indigenous Australians compared with the rest of the population, although less so than might be expected, given the size of the gap in health outcomes. Because of the relatively low incomes of Indigenous people, this pattern of higher spending was seen as an indication of greater public expenditures on poor people rather than on rich, as notions of equity would suggest is appropriate.

While it has not been possible to distinguish public from private spending in the present study, it has been possible, using 1995 NHS data, to be more discriminating about the relationship between overall expenditure and income status. For the first time, total spending on Indigenous and non-Indigenous people in equivalent income groups is estimated. This reveals that no significant difference exists between total expenditure on Indigenous and non-Indigenous Australians in the respective income quintiles. However, if hospital expenditure is excluded, then Indigenous expenditure is significantly lower for respective income groups. That is, controlling for income, Indigenous expenditure (other than on hospitals) is much lower than for other Australians. Given the lack of any discernible change to the low health status of Indigenous Australians during the 1990s, this supports, and even strengthens, the thrust of the Deeble et al. (1998) argument that an inverse care law applies—to those most in need, the least is given.

Of additional interest is the finding that relatively well-off Indigenous Australians, with presumably adequate access to (personal) resources, do not perceive their health to be any better than do lower-income Indigenous people. The proportion reporting fair to poor health status in the NHS did not vary significantly across income quintiles; just as in the NATSIS, having a long-term condition was found to be independent of income. This pattern contrasts sharply with that observed for the non-Indigenous population, for whom self-reported health status clearly improves with equivalent income. Why should relatively well-off Indigenous people consider their health to be on a par with those who are relatively poor? Perhaps more to the point, why should Indigenous people differ so much from other Australians of equivalent income in their self-reported health status?

One possible factor underlying this is the fact that Indigenous people are significantly less likely to have utilised health services in the two weeks prior to the NHS, even after controlling for income. In other words, they are significantly less likely overall to utilise health services. While cultural factors may impinge on health service utilisation, the extent to which these may contribute to this result remains poorly understood.

The general thrust of social epidemiological research, however, is now focused on the socio-economic standing of individuals and groups within society as the key to understanding health outcomes (Berkman and Kawachi 2000: Marmot and Wilkinson 1999). In this context, and given the trajectory of Indigenous economic development since the 1960s, it is arguable that the present generation of Indigenous people in the upper income quintiles are far more likely than their non-Indigenous counterparts to have been exposed to the trifecta of low birthweight, poor nutrition and childhood disease that can reap such havoc in later life. As Eades (2000) puts it, from a life-course perspective a person's current physiological status can be seen as a marker of their past social position.

This idea that adult mortality and morbidity may be related to foetal and infant life is generally referred to as the Barker hypothesis, or the foetal–infant origins hypothesis (Barker 1994). In particular, it is proposed that diseases such as coronary heart, type 2 diabetes, central obesity and hypertension (all highly prevalent among Indigenous adults) originate through adaptations that the foetus makes to under-nutrition. While the longitudinal data required for testing this hypothesis are generally unavailable for Indigenous Australians, some research on Indigenous health is emerging which appears to lend weight to the hypothesis, although the role played by the range of other risk factors in determining health outcomes remains difficult to disentangle (Hoy et al. 1999).

It is certainly the case that the current generation of Indigenous adults experienced dramatic change in life circumstances over the second half of the twentieth century. Much of what was stressful in this process and likely to have engendered poor health outcomes is detailed in the findings of the *Royal Commission into Aboriginal Deaths in Custody and in the Report of the National Inquiry into the Separation of Aboriginal and Torres Strait Islander Children from their Families* (Commonwealth of Australia 1991; HREOC 1997). Elsewhere, Gray, Trompf and Houston (1991) have examined the health consequences of family dissolution. Such analyses provide the essential context for a life-course perspective on extant Indigenous health profiles, something that survey data capture only poorly at best. As Gray (1992: 113–16) points out, it is astonishing to note how little is known about the social precedents of Indigenous morbidity and mortality. This can only be achieved if survey approaches enable health-determining processes to be located in the context of the place of each individual within his or her family, household and community.

An alternative explanation to the Barker hypothesis is that current income is probably a poor proxy for socio-economic status among Indigenous people, and hence the usual relationship between income, health status and expenditure is unlikely to be strong. The underlying reason why income is a poor proxy for socio-economic status among Indigenous people is that they have been, and continue to be, socially excluded from mainstream society, irrespective of current income (Hunter 2000a, 2000b, 2001). Social exclusion, unlike income poverty, is an intrinsically dynamic concept, descriptive of a condition which develops over time after a prolonged social isolation and deprivation.[20] The ongoing social exclusion and racial discrimination in Australia means that having a high income might not reflect social status, which is intrinsically conditioned by historical factors and other people's perceptions. Such contentions are supported by the renowned Whitehall study of British civil servants, which demonstrated that relative deprivation (defined in psychosocial terms) and the accumulation of socially patterned exposures over the life course are important explanations of the correlation between income and health status (Marmot & Smith 1997).[21]

While the Barker hypothesis implies a need to concentrate health expenditure on mothers and babies, the social exclusion hypothesis emphasises the need for ongoing support from both the community and governments across the entire life cycle. One possible implication of both of these hypotheses (albeit for different reasons) is that it will take a long time to address the health deficits among Indigenous Australians.

Ultimately, of course, the lack of any association between income and health status may simply reflect poor data quality, both in terms of income and self-assessed health status. The fact that poor-quality data restrict what can be said with confidence about the relationship between health expenditure, income and health status for the Indigenous population has been a consistent theme throughout this report. For example, we are unable to directly estimate the relationship between government health expenditure and income. We are also forced to exclude from the analysis the 20 per cent of the Indigenous population who live in sparsely settled areas of Australia. Most importantly, conventional income measures appear riddled with measurement error, with many Indigenous families moving up and down the distribution depending upon which measure is adopted. Measurement error is itself a major factor working against identifying a systematic relationship between income and health input and outputs; indeed, even if it were possible, it would be folly to believe that any causal relationship could be established, given uncertainty about the accuracy of Indigenous income status. Future research needs to clarify the role of measurement error in Indigenous income, and hence identify the extent to which income status can be usefully applied as an instrument for policy analysis.

As pointed out many times in the past, the collection of more reliable data is an essential prerequisite to improved analysis of equity issues in regard to health expenditure and health outcomes. From the analysis of NHS data it appears that improved reliability will depend on two developments—a larger augmented sample adequate to the task, and a reduction in non-sampling error in sparsely settled areas. While these improvements do not in themselves guarantee the quality of the data, they should increase the power of the analysis to discern whether the differences (and similarities) between Indigenous and other Australians in this paper are real or apparent.

Appendix A. Construction of utilisation rates using the 1995 National Health Survey

This appendix provides detailed definitions of each medical service and how the utilisation rates were calculated from the 1995 NHS. The question numbers refer to the numbering on the questionnaire as presented in the ABS *1995 National Health Survey Data Reference Pack*.

- **Hospital visits as an admitted patient:** Respondents were asked about visits to a hospital for their own health in the previous two weeks. Admitted hospital patients are those visiting a day clinic for minor surgery or diagnostic tests other than an x-ray, and hospitals other than as an outpatient or emergency patient. NHS Q508, Q509, Q510, Q511, Q512, Q513.

- **Hospital visits as a non-admitted patient:** Respondents were asked about visits to a hospital for their own health in the previous two weeks. Non-admitted hospital visits include: visits to the outpatients section of a hospital; and visits to a casualty or emergency ward of a hospital. NHS Q501, Q502, Q504, Q505, Q506.

- **Prescription medication:** Respondents were asked about medications they had used in the previous two weeks (vitamins and minerals are explicitly excluded). The respondent was then asked to get out the medications, and the names of all medications were then recorded. The respondent was then asked whether a prescription was needed to get each medication (up to a maximum of seven medications). If a prescription was needed then it was classified as a prescription medication. NHS Q605, Q606, Q608, Q614, Q625, Q636, Q647, Q658, Q669, Q680.

- **Non-prescription medication (see discussion for prescription medications):** Defined as a medication for which a prescription was not needed. NHS Q605, Q606, Q608, Q614, Q625, Q636, Q647, Q658, Q669, Q680.

- **Other health professionals**: includes acupuncturist, audiologist/audiometrist, chiropractor, chemist, chiropodist/podiatrist, dietician/nutritionist, herbalist, hypnotherapist, naturopath, nurse, optician/optometrist, osteopath, occupational therapist, physiotherapist/hydrotherapist, psychologist, social worker/welfare officer, speech therapist/pathologist, other. NHS Q520, Q521.

- **General practitioner and specialist:** excludes consultations during hospital and day clinic visits. NHS Q515, Q516.

Appendix B. Distribution of health expenditure by equivalent income

Table B.1   Per capita income, Indigenous

Quintile	Number in sample	Number with zero health	Number with expenditure of $1–1000	Number with expenditure of more than $1000	Maximum health expenditure
1	777	505	256	16	8365
2	279	136	136	7	9147
3	230	128	99	3	9137
4	165	80	82	3	4173
5	87	40	46	1	1947

Table B.2   Per capita income, non-Indigenous

Quintile	Number in sample	Number with zero health	Number with expenditure of $1–1000	Number with expenditure of more than $1000	Maximum health expenditure
1	9814	5009	4718	87	10059
2	9752	4519	5136	97	10315
3	10054	4496	5475	83	8922
4	9881	4335	5471	75	9280
5	10128	4590	5485	53	5987

Table B.3   Henderson equivalence scale, Indigenous

Quintile	Number in sample	Number with zero health	Number with expenditure of $1–1000	Number with expenditure of more than $1000	Maximum health expenditure
1	636	388	231	17	5516
2	408	247	154	7	9147
3	248	128	117	3	1964
4	149	71	76	2	4173
5	97	55	41	1	2060

Table B.4   Henderson equivalence scale, non-Indigenous

Quintile	Number in sample	Number with zero health	Number with expenditure of $1–1000	Number with expenditure of more than $1000	Maximum health expenditure
1	8505	3836	4570	99	10 120
2	8595	4018	4498	79	10 315
3	9001	4186	4736	79	8922
4	9257	4341	4860	56	7182
5	9696	4223	5414	59	9280

Table B.5   New OECD equivalence scale, Indigenous

Quintile	Number in sample	Number with zero health	Number with expenditure of $1–1000	Number with expenditure of more than $1000	Maximum health expenditure
1	658	406	235	17	5516
2	380	218	154	8	9147
3	256	145	110	1	1964
4	162	78	81	3	4173
5	82	42	39	1	1947

Table B.6   New OECD equivalence scale, non-Indigenous

Quintile	Number in sample	Number with zero health	Number with expenditure of $1–1000	Number with expenditure of more than $1000	Maximum health expenditure
1	9476	4486	4888	102	10 120
2	9616	4494	5032	90	10 315
3	9957	4654	5225	78	8912
4	10 384	4676	5644	64	7923
5	10 196	4639	5496	61	9280

Table B.7   Raw family income, Indigenous

Quintile	Number in sample	Number with zero health	Number with expenditure of $1–1000	Number with expenditure of more than $1000	Maximum health expenditure
1	446	249	187	10	9137
2	486	291	180	15	9147
3	309	178	129	2	1964
4	177	102	72	3	4173
5	120	69	51	0	419

Table B.8   Raw family income, non-Indigenous

Quintile	Number in sample	Number with zero health	Number with expenditure of $1–1000	Number with expenditure of more than $1000	Maximum health expenditure
1	9372	4546	4732	94	10120
2	9466	4419	4959	88	10315
3	9719	4490	5144	85	8922
4	10113	4556	5498	59	7923
5	10054	4520	5475	59	9280

Appendix C. Estimates of cost per medical service

This appendix presents the information on the average costs of medical services which is used in conjunction with the NHS 1995 to produce the estimates of per capita health expenditure. These estimates have been made using a variety of administrative and survey data sources by the AIHW. CAEPR has taken these estimates as given. CAEPR was provided with no information on the standard errors of these estimates or with enough information to allow the standard errors to be calculated.

Table C.1   Cost per day in hospital for admitted patients

	Male		Female	
	Non-Indigenous	Indigenous	Non-Indigenous	Indigenous
	$	$	$	$
Male				
0 to 4 years	743	732	724	708
5 to 9 years	892	791	900	786
10 to 14 years	861	783	831	757
15 to 19 years	764	719	710	577
20 to 24 years	627	560	683	567
25 to 29 years	624	580	675	591
30 to 34 years	631	576	683	584
35 to 39 years	693	611	702	633
40 to 44 years	714	693	695	620
45 to 49 years	692	484	688	665
50 to 54 years	733	565	701	616
55 to 59 years	755	658	699	613
60 to 64 years	720	567	707	594
65 to 69 years	733	588	685	473
70 to 74 years	690	558	661	544
75+ years	587	478	531	461
Total	678	621	640	607

Note: Acute patient costs for public and private hospitals are calculated using state DRG weights and are based on 1997–98 hospital data. Medical costs for private patients are not included. 1998–99 dollars. Expenditure is calculated using the Australian Refined (AR) system of diagnosis related groups (DRGs). Each AR-DRG represents a class of patients with similar clinical conditions requiring similar hospital services. Data were supplied to the AIHW by the state and territory health authorities, and by the Department of Veterans' Affairs for the hospitals it operated in NSW. Data were of two main types. The first, collated by AIHW as the National Public Hospital Establishments Database, included information about public hospitals, their resources, expenditure and revenue. The second type, collated as the National Hospital Morbidity Database, was patient-level data on the diagnoses and other characteristics of admitted patients in both public and private hospitals, and on the hospital care they received.

Table C.2   Out-of-hospital specialist services, cost per service, 1998–99

	Benefit paid ($)		Out of pocket expenditure ($)	
	Males	Females	Males	Females
Indigenous				
0–44	58	56	14	14
45+	51	51	11	11
Total	54	53	12	12
Non-Indigenous				
00–04	53	53	12	12
05–14	53	53	12	12
15–24	53	53	12	12
25–34	53	53	12	12
35–44	53	53	12	12
45–54	53	53	12	12
55–64	53	53	12	12
65–74	53	53	12	12
75+	53	53	12	12
Total	53	53	12	12

Note: Estimated using a combination of Medicare data and data from the Beach survey of general practitioners.

Table C.3   Out-of-hospital GP services, cost per service, 1998–99

	Benefit paid ($)		Out of pocket expenditure ($)	
	Males	Females	Males	Females
Indigenous				
00–04	75	62	7	6
05–14	32	30	3	3
15–24	26	60	2	5
25–34	49	87	4	9
35–44	54	83	5	9
45–54	85	94	10	12
55–64	85	147	8	13
65–74	123	144	6	6
75+	170	134	6	4
Total	50	68	5	7

Table C.3 Out-of-hospital GP services, cost per service, 1998–99 (continued)

	Benefit paid ($)		Out of pocket expenditure ($)	
	Males	Females	Males	Females
Non-Indigenous				
00–04	156	145	14	13
05–14	71	73	6	7
15–24	66	118	6	10
25–34	76	138	7	15
35–44	86	133	9	15
45–54	103	152	12	19
55–64	145	184	14	16
65–74	200	228	9	10
75+	216	314	7	9
Total	105	150	9	13

Note: Estimated using a combination of Medicare data and data from the Beach survey of general practitioners.

Table C.4 Prescription medications

	Benefit paid ($)		Out of pocket expenditure ($)	
	Males	Females	Males	Females
Males				
0–4	37.24	5.2	22.37	4.2
5–14	39.95	2.4	22.60	2.2
15–24	42.51	2.1	25.75	1.5
25–34	43.19	2.4	21.02	4.6
35–44	40.33	3.2	26.85	3.7
45–54	38.66	4.4	26.02	6.7
55–64	40.83	9.0	29.70	11.9
65–74	34.23	18.5	29.60	17.6
75+	21.48	27.1	27.87	10.1
Total	35.16	5.7	24.74	3.8

Table C.4   Prescription medications (continued)

| | Benefit paid ($) | | Out of pocket expenditure ($) | |
	Males	Females	Males	Females
Females				
0–4	35.52	5.0	19.79	4.2
5–14	36.67	2.6	21.29	1.7
15–24	43.74	4.0	29.13	2.8
25–34	44.39	4.3	24.14	5.4
35–44	41.03	4.6	26.92	5.4
45–54	41.62	6.2	26.79	7.8
55–64	40.55	12.6	30.70	15.5
65–74	33.10	22.8	35.30	12.0
75+	26.58	27.9	25.99	15.9
Total	36.09	8.0	26.10	4.6

Note: Estimated using a combination of administrative data on prescription medications and data from the Beach survey of general practitioners.

It was not possible to disaggregate costs for all medical service types. The following estimates were only available on an Australian-wide basis:

- *Non-admitted patients in public non-psychiatric hospitals*: For this medical service type there is only an Australia-wide estimate. The average cost per non-admitted patient is $95.64.

- *Over-the-counter medications*: For this medical service type there is only an Australia-wide estimate. The average cost per over-the-counter medication is $11.46.

- *Other health professionals*: For this medical service type there is only an Australia-wide estimate. The average cost per visit to another health professional is $61.24.

Appendix D. Method for estimation of standard errors and confidence intervals

With the exception of analysis of Table 5.1, all the standard errors in this paper are based on the 'jackknife method', which calculates the effect of each unit on the estimate. If there are n units in the sample, then n estimates are calculated from the sample where a single different unit is removed each time from the total sample. The variance estimate is then based on the difference between these estimates and the estimate obtained from the total sample (Wonnacott & Wonnacott 1984:250–1). The advantage of this method is that, even if the original estimate of variance is slightly biased (but asymptotically unbiased), the jackknife method will often eliminate the bias and produce consistent estimates of standard errors.

Given that jackknife errors were not obtained for the estimates of the proportion of the sample without health expenditure (Table 5.1), it is possible to derive some using the conventional binomial formula and adjusting for a design effect. That is, in order to account for the fact that the NHS is a complex sample rather than a simple random sample, the standard errors from the binomial formula need to be adjusted by a design effect.

The design effect was estimated as the factor by which the binomial standard errors must be scaled up to equate them with the (consistent) jackknife estimates of standard errors. This was done for both Indigenous and non-Indigenous population using the Table 6.2 jackknife estimates as the benchmark. For example, the jackknife estimates of the standard errors in that table were divided by the binomial estimates to derive a design effect specifically for all the estimates in Table 5.1.

Approximation of standard errors using the binomial formula and a design effect

Under simple random sampling (SRS), the estimate of variance of a proportion is given by

$$\hat{Var}_{SRS}(\hat{p}) = \frac{1}{n}(1 - \frac{n}{N})\hat{p}(1-\hat{p})$$

B1:

p = esitmate of proportion

n = sample size

$\hat{Var}_{SRS}$ = estimate of the variance of the estimate of proportion, assuming SRS

N = sample size

For large N, as in our case, we can simplify this to:

$$\hat{Var}_{SRS}(\hat{p}) = \frac{1}{n}\hat{p}(1-\hat{p})$$

B2:

Under a complex desigh the variance of the estimate can be estimated by:

$$\hat{Var}_{complex}(\hat{p}) = deff \times \hat{Var}_{SRS}$$ (B3)

$$= deff \frac{1}{n}\hat{p}(1-\hat{p})$$

where *deff*=design effect

As indicated above, the design effect was calculated using the jackknife estimates for Table 6.2 and then used to scale up the estimated variances for a simple random sample using equation B3.

Combining standard errors for confidence intervals

This section provides a methodology of how to calculate standard errors for a difference in two random variables. From basic statistical theory, the variance (Var) of a difference is:

$$Var(x-y) = Var(x) + Var(y) - 2Cov(x,y)$$ (B4)

Ignoring the co-variance (Cov) term, or rather assuming it is positive and bounding it below by 0, yields formula (B5):

$$se(x-y) = \sqrt{se(x)^2 + se(y)^2}$$ (B5)

While this formula is theoretically valid under SRS only (i.e. assuming independence), it is widely used in publications based on complex household sample designs, such as the *Labour Force Status*. To test its validity under these circumstances a quick empirical study was undertaken using Indigenous data from the 1994 Australian Housing Survey (see ABS 2001 for details).

An alternative, more conservative approach, is to bound the co-variance using a Cauchy-Schwarz inequality (i.e. $Cov(x,y) =< se(x)se(y)$), which leads to the formula:

$$se(x-y) =< se(x) + se(y)$$ (B6)

Equation B5 worked quite well in ABS (2001), while equation B6 was found to overestimate standard errors, but not drastically. While the co-variance cannot always be neglected, the ABS study provides no evidence against the use of equation B5 in surveys with Indigenous components. Also, equation B6 may not be a good alternative as, being an upper bound, it will always overestimate the true variation. Given the ABS previous experience, the confidence intervals and inferences in this paper use the formula in equation B5.

Notes

1. The health–social status correlation is hypothesised to occur because: (1) social position impacts health through access to health care, nutrition, working conditions etc; (2) health determines social status (the health selection hypothesis); or (3) common factors determine both social position and health (a variation of the health selection hypothesis)—that is, the social epidemiology literature tends to discount the health selection hypothesis.

2. Sparsely settled areas are defined as statistical local areas (SLAs) where the dwelling density for the SLA as a whole is less than 57 dwellings per 100 square kilometres.

3. The standardised morbidity ratio is equal to hospital separations identified as Indigenous divided by expected separations based on all-Australia rates.

4. The rationale behind the use of equivalence scales is based on the simple fact that, for example, a six-person family can usually live more cheaply than six single people can. As a result of economies of scale, a six-person family does not need six times the resources of one person to reach the same welfare. That is, an additional family member does not cause a proportionate increase in expenditure on, say, heating or housing.

5. Sensitivity testing to a variety of equivalence scales is a common practice in research (Burniaux et al. 1998). For example, Atkinson (1995) considered income inequality using raw family/household income (that is, no adjustment for family size—an 'equivalence scale elasticity' of zero) and per capita income ('equivalence scale elasticity' of one). They found that the level of income inequality was higher with these assumptions than when measured using the square root of the number of people in the family ('equivalence scale elasticity' of 0.5). The equivalence scale elasticities between zero and one cover the majority of possible assumptions about household costs, from there being no extra cost to additional persons living in the household to there being no economies of scale in people living in a household.

6. To facilitate the exposition, this paper equates 'family' with 'income unit' as defined by the ABS. Income unit is the social grouping across which the ABS assesses that aggregate income is effectively shared.

7. The 1995 NHS data provides income data adjusted using a version of the simplified Henderson equivalence scales.

8. See Buhman et al. (1988) for a single parameter estimate of 'equivalence elasticities'. These elasticities provide a rough guide to what we have called economies of scale.

9. In an analysis of Indigenous housing disadvantage, Neutze, Sanders and Jones (1999: 45) found that high rates of home ownership in low-income groups were driven by the disproportionate numbers of retired persons in such groups.

10. 'Jackknifing' is a method used for estimating the standard errors of estimates obtained from complex sample surveys. The jackknife method involves repeated sampling from subsets of the sample data. The characteristics of the repeated sub-samples are used to estimate the variance over the entire data set – that is, the method calculates the effect of each unit on the estimate. If there are n units in the sample, then n estimates are calculated from the sample where a single different unit is removed each time from the total sample (Levy & Lemeshow 1999: 378).

11. Deeble et al. (1998) include the following medical services in their estimates of health expenditure by income group for the total Australian population: inpatient and outpatient hospital services; out-of-hospital GP and specialist medical services; allied health services; and prescribed drugs.

12. However, it was possible to present some statistics for Indigenous people from each quintile where the estimates were reasonably reliable. See Appendix B.

13. The cost per GP and specialist visit is estimated using data from the Bettering the Evaluation and Care of Health (BEACH) survey. The BEACH survey collects information from about 100 GPs a year and asks them about the details of the patients they treat (results in data on about 100 000 patient encounters per year). Information about the presenting problems of patients, diagnosis, and treatments prescribed and given is available. In addition sociodemographic characteristics of the patients, including whether patients are Aborigines or Torres Strait Islanders, are recorded.

14. For prescription medications which are listed on the PBS schedule, the share of the costs borne privately versus publicly depends upon the amount of the subsidy, whether or not the individual has a health care card, their income and the amount they have spent on prescription medications in the current year.

15. The estimate of the average per capita health expenditure for the non-Indigenous population implied by Table 2 differs to the overall estimate reported in a previous paragraph due to the omission of several individuals with very high levels of health expenditure which happen to have missing values for the income variables. This is also true for the estimates of expenditure by income reported in Tables 4.3 and 4.4.

16. The hospital services data excluded from the estimates are: number of visits to a hospital; number of visits to casualty/emergency; number of visits to outpatients; and number of visits to day clinic. As indicated above, these are low frequency events which are unlikely to have occurred in the previous two weeks and hence their exclusion should enhance the reliability of the estimates.

17. That is, health expenditure is highly skewed. A recent US study shows that, in a year, 27% of the expenditure is by 1% of users, and 97% by 50% of users (Berk & Monheit 2001). Of that top 1%, 46% are elderly.

18. In addition approximately half of the original sample were asked to complete a written supplement comprising the Short Form-36 (SF-36) health status questionnaire. The SF-36 is a well-known measure of general health and well-being; it produces scores

for eight dimensions of health. Selection into this 'treatment' group was based on the random assignment of blocks within census districts. Approximately 30% of the Indigenous sample was administered the SF-36. Given the small Indigenous sample, it is not possible to make use of the SF-36 in a comparison of the health status of the Indigenous and non-Indigenous population.

19. The SF-36 is a well-known measure of general health and well-being which produces scores for eight dimensions of health in the reporting of long-term health questions. It has been extensively validated for many samples from many countries (Ware, Snow & Gandek 1993).

20. In economic terms, poverty is a static concept defined by whether an individual, family or household has sufficient income at a particular point of time.

21. Social, economic and political factors have an important influence on health and longevity, but the social position and lifestyle patterns of individuals only partially explain ill health. Psychosocial factors, such as a sense of isolation, deprivation or loss of control, are also important (Marmot 2000). Another factor is that relatively high income may be a relatively recent phenomenon for Indigenous people and, consequently, it may be difficult for these newly wealthy people to adjust to their changing circumstances. For example, compared with those experiencing no significant organisational change, men exposed to major changes in their workplace demonstrated increases in all self-reported morbidity measures, including health ratings of average or worse, adverse sleep patterns, long-standing illness, mean number of symptoms in the previous fortnight, blood pressure, and body mass index (Ferrie et al. 1998). In the Indigenous context, the pressure of frequently being the first Indigenous person in an organisation adds extra stress into the working environment.

References

Altman, J.C. and Hunter, B. 1998. 'Indigenous poverty', in R. Fincher and J. Nieuwenhuysen (eds), *Australian Poverty: Then and Now*, Melbourne University Press, Melbourne.

Altman, J.C., Hunter, B., Smith, D.E. and Taylor, J. 1997. Indigenous Australians and the National Survey of Living Standards, Unpublished report to the Department of Social Security, CAEPR, ANU, Canberra.

Atkinson, A.B., Rainwater, L. and Smeeding, T. 1995. 'Income distribution in OECD countries: evidence from the Luxembourg income study', *Social Policy Studies No. 18*, OECD, Paris.

Australian Bureau of Statistics (ABS) 1996. *Health of Indigenous Australians: National Aboriginal and Torres Strait Islander Survey*, Cat. no. 4395.0, ABS, Canberra.

Australian Bureau of Statistics 1998. *Experimental Estimates of the Aboriginal and Torres Strait Islander Population*, ABS Cat. no. 3230.0, ABS, Canberra.

Australian Bureau of Statistics 1999. *1995 National Health Survey: Aboriginal and Torres Strait Islander Results*, Cat. no. 4806.0, ABS, Canberra.

Australian Bureau of Statistics 2000a. *Deaths, 1999*, Cat. no. 3302.0, ABS, Canberra.

Australian Bureau of Statistics 2000b. *Housing and Infrastructure in Aboriginal and Torres Strait Islander Communities Australia 1999*, Cat. no. 4710.0, ABS, Canberra.

Australian Bureau of Statistics 2000c. *Labour Force Characteristics of Aboriginal and Torres Strait Islander Australians: Experimental Estimates from the Labour Force Survey*, Cat. no. 6287.0, ABS, Canberra.

Australian Bureau of Statistics 2001. Estimating the standard error (SE) of the movement in unemployment rate for estimates in the Labour Force Characteristics of Aboriginal and Torres Strait Islander Australians, Unpublished paper, ABS, Canberra.

Australian Bureau of Statistics and Australian Institute of Health and Welfare (AIHW) 1999. *The Health and Welfare of Australia's Aboriginal and Torres Strait Islander Peoples*, Cat. no. 4704.0, ABS, Canberra.

Barker D.J.P. 1994. *Mothers, Babies and Diseases in Later Life*, BMJ Publishing Group, London.

Bartlett, B. and Legge, D. 1994. 'Supporting Aboriginal Health Services: a program for the Commonwealth Department of Human Services and Health', *NCEPH Working Paper No. 34*, National Centre for Epidemiology and Population Health, ANU, Canberra.

Berk, M. and Monheit, A. 2001. 'The concentration of health care expenditures revisited', *Health Affairs*, 20 (2): 9–32.

Berkman, L. F. and Kawachi, I. 2000. *Social Epidemiology*, OUP, New York.

Buhman, B., Rainwater, L., Schmaus, G. and Smeeding, T. M. 1988. 'Equivalence scales, well-being, inequality, and poverty: Sensitivity estimates across ten countries using the Luxembourg Income Study (LIS) database', *The Review of Income and Wealth*, 34 (2): 115–42.

Burniaux, J., Dang, T., Fore, D., Forster, M., D'Ercole, M. and Oxley, H. 1998. 'Income distribution and poverty in selected OECD countries', *Economics Department Working Paper No. 189*, OECD, Paris.

Commonwealth of Australia 1991. *Royal Commission into Aboriginal Deaths in Custody*, vol. 4, (Commissioner E. Johnson), AGPS, Canberra.

Commonwealth of Australia 1999. The National Indigenous Housing Guide: Improving the Living Environment for Safety, Health and Sustainability, Unpublished report, Commonwealth, State and Territory Housing Ministers Working Group on Indigenous Housing, Canberra.

Cunningham, J. and Beneforti, M. 2000. *Occasional Paper: Hospital Statistics, Aboriginal and Torres Strait Islander Australians 1997–98*, ABS, Canberra.

Cunningham, J. and Mackerras, D. 1998. *Occasional Paper: Overweight and Obesity, Indigenous Australians*, ABS, Canberra.

Cunningham, J. and Paradies, Y. 2000. *Occasional Paper: Mortality of Aboriginal and Torres Strait Islander Australians, 1997*, Cat. no. 3315.0, ABS, Canberra.

Cunningham, J., Sibthorpe, B. and Anderson, I. 1997. *Occasional Paper: Self-Assessed Health Status, Indigenous Australians*, Cat. no. 4707.0, ABS, Canberra.

Daly, A. and Smith, D.E. 1998a. 'Indigenous sole parents: welfare dependence and work opportunities', *Australian Bulletin of Labour*, 24 (1): 47–66.

Daly, A.E. and Smith, D.E. 1998b. 'The continuing disadvantage of Indigenous sole parents: a preliminary analysis of 1996 Census data', *CAEPR Discussion Paper No. 153*, CAEPR, ANU, Canberra.

De Vos, K. and Zaidi, M.A. 1997. 'Equivalence scale sensitivity of poverty statistics for the member states of the European Community', *Review of Income and Wealth*, 43 (3): 319–33.

Deeble, J., Mathers, C., Smith, L., Goss, J., Webb, R. and Smith, V. 1998. *Expenditures on Health Services for Aboriginal and Torres Strait Islander People*, Commonwealth Department of Health and Family Services, Canberra.

Eades, S.J. 2000. 'Reconciliation, social equity and Indigenous health', *Medical Journal of Australia*, 172: 468–69.

Ferrie, J. E., Shipley, M. J., Marmot, M. G., Stansfeld, S. et al. 1998. 'The health effects of major organisational change and job insecurity', *Social Science and Medicine*, 46 (2): 243–254.

Gray, A. 1992. 'Health and housing in Aboriginal and Torres Strait Islander communities', in J.C. Altman (ed.), *A National Survey of Indigenous Australians: Options and Implications*, CAEPR Research Monograph No. 3, CAEPR, ANU, Canberra.

Gray, A. and Broughton, B. 2001. 'Education and health behaviour of Indigenous Australians: Evidence from the 1994 National Aboriginal and Torres Strait Islander Survey (NATSIS)', *Occasional Paper No. 3*, Cooperative Research Centre for Aboriginal and Tropical Health, Darwin.

Gray, A.P., Trompf, P. and Houston, S. 1991. 'The decline and rise of Aboriginal families', in J. Reid and P. Trompf (eds), *The Health of Aboriginal Australia*, Harcourt Brace Jovanovich, Sydney.

Gray, B. 1997. 'Indigenous data quality in the National Health Survey 1995: Analysis of selected questions from the unedited, unweighted file', *ABS Internal Discussion Paper 97/1*, National Centre for Aboriginal and Torres Strait Islander Statistics, ABS, Darwin.

Guobao, W., Richardson, S. and Travers, P. 1996. 'Multiple deprivation in rural China', *Working Paper No. 96/1*, Chinese Economy Research Centre, University of Adelaide, Adelaide.

Henderson, R.F. (Chairman) 1975. *'Commission of Inquiry into Poverty: Poverty in Australia*, First Main Report, Australian Government Publishing Service, Canberra.

Hogg, R. S. 1990. 'Insights into Aboriginal mortality in Western New South Wales', in A. Gray (ed.), *A Matter of Life and Death: Contemporary Aboriginal Mortality*, Aboriginal Studies Press, Canberra.

Hogg, R. S. 1992. 'Indigenous mortality: placing Australian Aboriginal mortality within a broader context', *Social Science and Medicine*, 35 (3): 335–46.

Hoy, W.E., Rees, M., Kile, E., Mathews, J.D. and Wang, Z. 1999. 'A new dimension to the Barker hypothesis: low birthweight and susceptibility to renal disease', *Kidney International*, 56 (3): 1072–7.

Human Rights and Equal Opportunity Commission (HREOC) 1997. *Bringing them Home: Report of the National Inquiry into the Separation of Aboriginal and Torres Strait Islander Children from their Families*, HREOC, Sydney.

Hunter, B.H. 1999. 'Three nations, not one: Indigenous and other Australian poverty', *CAEPR Working Paper No. 1*, CAEPR, ANU, Canberra, available on the WWW at http:online.anu.edu.au/caepr/.

Hunter, B.H. 2000a. 'The social costs of Indigenous unemployment', *Economic and Labour Relations Review*, 11 (2): 213–32.

Hunter, B.H. 2000b. 'Social exclusion, social capital and Indigenous Australians: Measuring the social costs of unemployment', *CAEPR Discussion Paper No. 204*, CAEPR, ANU, Canberra.

Hunter, B.H. 2001. 'Tackling poverty among Indigenous Australians', in R. Fincher and P. Saunders (eds), *Creating Unequal Futures*, Allen and Unwin, Sydney.

Hunter, B.H. and Smith, D.E. 2000. 'Surveying mobile populations: lessons from recent longitudinal surveys of Indigenous Australians', *CAEPR Discussion Paper No. 203*, CAEPR, ANU, Canberra.

Hunter, B.H., Kennedy, S. and Smith, D. 2001. 'Sensitivity of Australian income distributions to choice of equivalence scale: Exploring some parameters of Indigenous incomes', *CAEPR Working Paper No. 11*, CAEPR, ANU, Canberra, available on the WWW at http://online.anu.edu.au/caepr/.

Jones, R. 1999. 'Indigenous Housing 1996 Census Analysis', Aboriginal and Torres Strait Islander Commission, Canberra.

Kawachi, I., Kennedy, B.P. and Wilkinson, R.G. 1999. *The Society and Population Health Reader: Income Inequality and Health*, New Press, New York.

Kunitz, S.J. 1990. 'Public policy and mortality among indigenous populations of Northern America and Australasia', *Population and Development Review*, 16 (4): 647–72.

Levy, P. S. and Lemeshow, S. 1999. *Sampling of Populations: Methods and Applications*, John Wiley and Sons, New York.

Marmot, M. 2000. 'Social determinants of health: from observation to policy', *Medical Journal of Australia*, 172 (8): 379–82.

Marmot, M.G. and Smith, G.D. 1997. 'Socio-economic differentials in health: The contribution of the Whitehall studies', *Journal of Health Psychology*, 2 (3): 283–96.

Marmot, M. and Wilkinson, R.G. 1999. *Social Determinants of Health*, OUP, New York.

McDermott, R.A., Plant, A.J. and Mooney, G. 1996. 'Has access to hospital improved for Aborigines in the Northern Territory?', *Australian and New Zealand Journal of Public Health*, 20 (6): 589–93.

National Centre for Epidemiology and Population Health (NCEPH) 2000. *Commonwealth Grants Commission (CGC) Indigenous Funding Inquiry, Submission No. IfI/SUB/0025*, CGC, Canberra.

National Health Strategy (NHS) 1992. 'Enough to make you sick: How income and environment affect health', *National Health Strategy Research Paper No.12*, Melbourne.

Neutze, M., Sanders, W. and Jones, G. 1999. 'Public Expenditure on Services for Indigenous People Education, Employment, Health and Housing', *Discussion Paper No. 24*, The Australia Institute, Canberra.

Ruben, A.R. and Walker, A.C. 1995. 'Malnutrition among rural Aboriginal children in the Top End of the Northern Territory', *The Medical Journal of Australia*, 162 (8): 400–03.

Saunders, P. 1994. *Welfare and Inequality*, Cambridge University Press, Cambridge.

Sibthorpe, B. 1988. 'All our People are Dyin': Diet and Stress in an Urban Aboriginal Community, unpublished PhD thesis, Anthropology Department, ANU, Canberra.

Taylor, J. and Hunter, B. 1998. *The Job Still Ahead: Economic Costs of Continuing Indigenous Employment Disparity*, Office of Public Affairs, Aboriginal and Torres Strait Islander Commission, Canberra.

Torzillo, P. and Kerr, C. 1991. 'Contemporary issues in Aboriginal public health', in J. Reid and P. Trompf (eds), *The Health of Aboriginal Australia*, Harcourt Brace Jovanovich, Sydney.

Travers, P. and Richardson, S. 1993. *Living Decently: Material Well-being in Australia*, OUP, Melbourne.

Ware, J.,K., Snow, J. and Gandek, B.1993. *SF-36 Health Survey Manual and Interpretation Guide*, The Health Institute, New England Medical Centre, Boston, Massachusetts.

Wonnacott, T.H. and Wonnacott, R.J. 1984. *Introductory Statistics for Business and Economics*, John Wiley & Sons, New York.

CAEPR Research Monograph Series

18.   *Ngukurr at the Millennium: A Baseline Profile for Social Impact Planning in South-East Arnhem Land*, J. Taylor, J. Bern, and K.A. Senior, 2000.

19.   *Aboriginal Nutrition and the Nyirranggulung Health Strategy in Jawoyn Country*, J. Taylor and N. Westbury, 2000.

20.   *The Indigenous Welfare Economy and the CDEP Scheme*, F. Morphy and W. Sanders (eds), 2001.

21.   *Health Expenditure, Income and Health Status among Indigenous and Other Australians,* M.C. Gray, B.H. Hunter and J. Taylor, 2002.

For information on CAEPR Discussion Papers and Research Monographs please contact:

Publication Sales, Centre for Aboriginal Economic Policy Research, The Australian National University, Canberra, ACT, 0200

Telephone: 02–6125 8211
Facsimile: 02–6125 9730

Information on CAEPR abstracts and summaries of all CAEPR print publications and those published electronically can be found at the following WWW address:

http://online.anu.edu.au/caepr/

www.ingramcontent.com/pod-product-compliance
Lightning Source LLC
Chambersburg PA
CBHW061222270326
41927CB00022B/3470